Keto Diet Lifestyle:

Regain Confidence with the Ultimate Beginners Ketogenic Manual for Healthy Weight Loss Including 5+ Golden Rules and Recipes to Reboot Your Metabolism

Patrick H. Smith

Table of Contents

Intermittent Fasting Guide for Beginners:

Your Ultimate 5+ Techniques for Healthy Detox, Weight loss with Fat Burn Secrets to reset Metabolism and Heal Your Body Including also Keto Diet principles

By Patrick H. Smith

Table of Contents

Keto Diet Lifestyle:

By Patrick H. Smith

Disclaimer

The information listed by the author in this book is not intended, by the author or the publisher, to diagnose or treat any illnesses or diseases. The information herein is meant to provide helpful background and understanding of the topics and their theories. For diagnosis or treatment of any disease, illness, or medical problem, please contact a medical professional in that field. Neither the publisher nor the author is responsible or liable for any allergy or medical needs not addressed or exacerbated by the use of the information herein. No information in these pages should be construed as medical, legal, or psychological advice or instruction. All data is provided for informational purposes and does not constitute endorsement on behalf of the author or publisher.

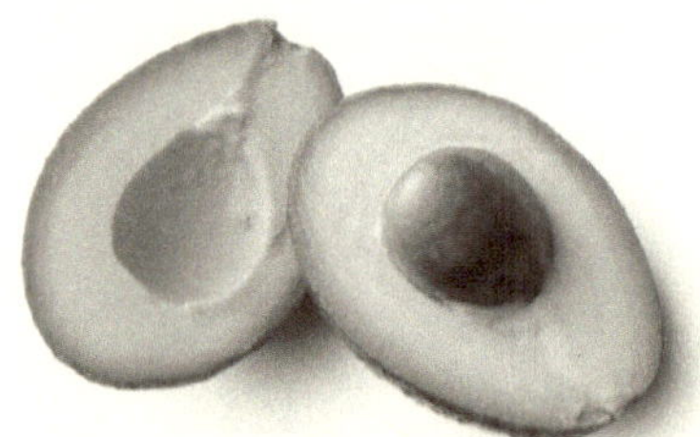

(Avocado)

Introduction

Keto Diet Lifestyle: Regain Confidence with the Ultimate Beginners Ketogenic Manual for Healthy Weight Loss Including 5+ Golden Rules and Recipes to Reboot Your Metabolism is brought to you by Patrick H. Smith, an American author who specializes in nutrition, health, and fitness. Patrick is a coach and motivational speaker with a passion for sharing the best tips he's learned while maintaining a ketogenic diet with a busy working schedule.

One problem that has often been cited as the reason we can't seem to keep ourselves eating healthy foods, is because we're constantly running throughout the day. From the time we wake up, to the time we fall asleep, we are on a time crunch, and finding the time to make all our meals and snacks at home can take a lot of time we don't think we have in our day. As someone who is familiar with working on a busy schedule, who is familiar with having to make time in the middle of a hectic day, Patrick H. Smith is here to show us how we can get the best foods for us, even on a hectic schedule.

The following chapters will discuss many tools that you can use to get started on a ketogenic diet, while living your busy life around it. You'll get the best tips and tricks, delicious recipes, and the best-kept secrets about making this diet work for you. Get answers for the most common questions, solutions to the most common problems, and get the most valuable tips that will keep you going on a diet that is meant to help you feel better *for life.*

There is a wealth of resources on the subject of keto diets, and it can get a little bit overwhelming having to sift through all of it. All the legwork is done for you here in *Keto Diet: Regain Confidence with the Ultimate Beginners Ketogenic Manual for Healthy Weight Loss Including 5+ Golden Rules and Recipes to Reboot Your Metabolism.* All the most pertinent information, best tricks, and recipes have been compiled for you right here in one place. Search no more and finally get to work on enjoying your ketogenic diet and the many benefits it has to offer you!

.Chapter 1: What is the Ketogenic Diet?

The Ketogenic Diet, or keto for short, is a diet that has gained a lot of traction recently. There is a lot of buzz about it being a low-carb diet, that it helps people lose weight at a rapid pace, and that it is a somewhat easier diet to commit to than others that have been in the mainstream. There are a lot of specifics about the diet, however, that don't seem to make it to the forefront of the public eye. This book will outline everything there is to know about living on a ketogenic diet, what that means for you and your body, how best to keep to that sort of diet, and how it differs from and is similar to other diets.

In general, tracking the amounts of calories you eat on a daily basis isn't something that is done. Even rarer is tracking what the breakdown of nutrients in those calories is. This means that you would really have no way of knowing how many carbohydrates you're taking in, how much fat, how much protein, and what the balances is between these three macronutrients. Having a heavy concentration of carbohydrates in your body means that you'll be burning those to create energy that you'll use to get through your day.

It's helpful to think of your body as running on two basic modes when it comes to digestion and metabolism of nutrients. The first, and most common mode for the typical American diet, is running off of carbohydrates. These are metabolized into sugar, which is then turned into the energy your body uses to conduct all its necessary functions. The other mode is to run off of fat from the stores in your body, as well as in the food that you eat. When your body is running off of fat, your liver switches from producing insulin, to producing ketones. This is where we get the term "ketogenic," to describe this low-carb diet. It is also why it is such an effective, fat-burning diet.

The way to switch over to this second mode of digestion, is to give your body a dearth of carbohydrates to burn for energy. If there are no carbohydrates available for your body to burn, your system will kick into survival mode and switch to that other mode. All your energy will come from the fat you're eating, as well as the fat that your body has already stored away. This is the excess weight that many of us are striving to lose. By giving your body something to do with that excess fat in your body, it will burn much more quickly.

<u>What is Ketosis?</u>

When people talk about their progress with the keto diet, they often talk about "being in ketosis." This is the biological process that many dieters strive for, because it is the basis of the ketogenic diet, and it accelerates your progress with it. But what is it?

Simply put, it is that second mode of operating for your digestive system, that tells your body to burn fats for energy instead of sugars. This is a very simplified explanation of what is going on, and there are more intricacies to what your body is doing, but this is a foot in the door, so to speak, when working to understand that process.

Once your body has begun this process, you will find that you have more energy than you realized you lacked in the first place. This is due to the fact that fat burning is occurring around the clock, even when you're completely at rest or asleep. Your body shifts into this mode of using every bit of stored energy you have, to complete even the most basic functions your body needs to survive.

How Can Keto Help Me?

There are many things that a ketogenic diet can help to resolve. The nature of the diet is such that, if you're keeping to it properly, your body will begin to thrive. You will be eliminating things from your diet like processed foods and sugar. It is recommended that you eat natural foods that contain healthy fats and nutrients your body needs.

Keeping the body fed with natural, wholesome foods, removing the sugar dependency that most of us have, and increasing your energy levels are benefits we could all use. In addition to this, studies show us that there are several diseases, illnesses, and physical ailments that are caused by the foods that we eat and can be reversed by taking charge of and fixing our diets.

The keto diet works best when you eat plenty of natural vegetables while keeping your carbohydrates, fats, and protein within the proper ranges. We will go into more about what those ranges are and why it's imperative that you ensure you're keeping to them. While calorie counting is not the main focus of the keto diet, it is important to analyze what nutrients those calories contain. Calorie-counting apps are a great way to keep an eye on this, as they'll break down that makeup for you and show you exactly what you're eating.

One of the biggest benefits of doing a ketogenic diet is that you're eliminating things from your diet that have been proven to cause illness or health issues. There are many links between several different illnesses and foods that are high in chemical preservatives, additives, sweeteners, and carbohydrates. Illnesses like type 2 diabetes and heart disease are chief among them.

Let's take a look at some bullet points that highlight the benefits of keto:

- A more sustainable, higher energy level. That means you can do more in your waking hours, *without* crashing!
- Less dependency on sugar for energy or comfort
- Fewer cravings for foods that don't help your body
- No need to snack throughout the day
- Better, more restful sleep that leaves you feeling energized and ready to tackle the day
- Healthier lifestyle that allows you to keep the hobbies and activities you love
- A completely sustainable new lifestyle that doesn't depend on foods that are harmful to the body
- Reverse and avoid illnesses that can come about as a result of poor nutrition or diet
- Inevitable loss of excess body fat

As you learn more about what constitutes a ketogenic diet, you may find that it shares some similarities with other diets that are currently popular. Let's look through those diets and point out the things about them that are the most similar to keto.

Low-Carb

This is sort of a general regimen change that you may even automatically associate with keto these days. The principal behind low-carb is a rather simple one: eliminate bread and carb-heavy foods from your diet, lose weight.

This is a very shallow view of the principals behind keto and doesn't cover several other specifics that need to be in place for a truly ketogenic diet. Many people who are sticking to a low-carb regimen will often fill in their daily calories with a lot of dairy, red meat, and pork. While this does work for some, it's not the best way to go about achieving ketosis, and it's not the best way to go about avoiding some of the common bodily issues that can be caused by these types of foods.

We'll get into more about how the daily meals for a ketogenic diet should look, what they should contain, and how best to keep yourself looking and feeling healthier by the day. We'll show you exactly how your macronutrients should be balanced, as well as what the best sources are for those macronutrients. Let's take a look at the next item on our list.

Gluten-Free

These days, you will notice that a large percentage of the foods we buy have labels on them that declare they're gluten-free. Why is this? What is gluten? What is the gluten-free diet and why would it be beneficial for someone to adhere to it? Several years ago, gluten gained the status of a common allergen. Cases of wheat intolerance have grown in number over the past several years and people are doing their best to remove gluten from their everyday diets.

Gluten is a protein that is found specifically in wheat, barley, rye, and hybrids between those three. In people who are allergic to it, it can cause a wide range of symptoms that may go unnoticed by the patient until gluten is cut from their diet. In people who are not allergic to gluten, it is perfectly harmless. The only dietary need to stay away from gluten, other than an intolerance, would be to avoid bread and carbs altogether.

The most commonly known illness connected to gluten is Celiac disease, which is an illness that is only sensitive to gluten. It's actually an autoimmune disease that causes your system to attack your small intestine when there is gluten present. When ingested, the lining of the small intestine becomes inflamed, causing bloating, diarrhea, and other painful stomach issues. Those who suffer from this illness will find that once they cut this protein from their diet, digestion goes much more smoothly, and they have an easier time getting through the day.

Another part, or a sort of offshoot of Celiac disease is Dermatitis Herpetiformis, which alters the response that Celiac has. That autoimmune response of the system attacking the small intestine shifts to attack the skin. This means that after you eat gluten, you will notice painful rashes developing on the skin, which can sometimes be mistaken for severe acne. One of the largest telltale signs of DH is that the pattern of the rash is general symmetrical, so this is something to look for if you regularly consume gluten without even realizing what it's doing to your skin.

It is unclear at this time what prolonged exposure to gluten will do to someone with this autoimmune disease, outside of the symptoms they cause in the immediate term. Avoiding gluten is much easier these days than it has been previously, as there are so many options for replacing those grains that contain gluten.

The neat thing about keto is that it *is* gluten-free. Because it's your aim to cut out all carb-heavy items from your diet, you won't find that wheat (the source of gluten) will make its way into your diet anymore. Now, where keto and a gluten-free diet cease to overlap is that someone who is only trying to be gluten-free can use flour alternatives such as oats, rice, and other grains. On keto, we're simply eliminating the need for grains, so there is no replacement.

So, in short, the ketogenic diet *is* gluten-free, but a gluten-free is not necessarily ketogenic!

Paleo

Paleo, the paleolithic diet, the caveman diet, the hunter-gatherer diet, or the stone-age diet is a diet that utilizes a very unique criterion for its basis. Paleo is a diet that restricts what you can eat to what was available to hunter-gatherers up until about 10,000 years ago. This means lean meats, fish, vegetables, fruits, seeds, and nuts. This does not include things that only became available with the advent of farming such as dairy products, legumes, and grains.

The theory behind eating these types of foods and restricting ourselves to only what was available prior to 10,000 years ago, comes down to the quality of the foods we're taking in. It is theorized that the human body hasn't evolved since that time, and so our bodies are not meant to take on the types of foods that make up the modern diet. The theory that the human body isn't meant to ingest the types of foods that came about thanks to modernized farming, is known as the Discordance Hypothesis.

The theory is that because humans advanced their farming techniques so quickly and because so many new types of foods were introduced in the last 10,000 years, the human body hasn't been able to catch up. Thanks to this evolutionary misstep, we have an ever-growing obesity epidemic, more food-related illnesses being revealed as time goes on, and less overall health in the human species.

By sticking to the foods that made up the diets of our ancestors, we're giving the body only what it needs in order to create clean, pure energy for the body. We're not giving the body anything it can't tolerate, or anything with which it can create problems, excess fat, or disease. This does not, however, automatically translate to a ketogenic diet.

While Paleo is a diet that can help with a great many things, it is not a keto diet. There are some foods available on that diet that can kick and keep your body out of ketosis, which won't make you the fat-burning powerhouse that you can be with keto.

Atkins

Atkins was an incredibly popular low-carb, high-protein, high-fat diet. Dr. Robert Atkins came onto the market with his dietary products in 1989. In the 1990s, the diet gained much traction as the be all, end all to nutrition and weight loss. As far as low-carb diets went, The Atkins Diet became nearly synonymous. This is why today, when people hear about keto, they think about Atkins.

Now, the principal behind Atkins is that if you cut your carbs to nil, increase your protein intake beyond what you've eaten in the past, and eat a large amount of fat from foods like red met, pork, and dairy, you will lose weight. Your body will run off of all that fat and produce unrivaled results in terms of weight loss.

The drawbacks that have been discovered in the Atkins diet is that many of the dieters weren't introducing enough vegetables, healthy fats, or lean proteins into their diet. This had the unfortunate effect of increasing the risk of coronary diseases and events. Many dieters were focused on steak, butter, cream, bacon, and sugar-free dessert options like gelatin.

When doing the Atkins diet, it is ideal to take on mostly low-glycemic foods. Foods that do not spike your blood sugar level, and which do not stimulate insulin production in the body. This includes whole foods with little to no sugar, natural or otherwise, and with low carbohydrate or starch content. The theory here is, if you're eating foods that keep your blood sugar even, you won't ever experience crashes, binging behavior, or cravings.

Now how do keto and the Atkins diet differ if both diets call for low-glycemic foods, little to no carbs, and whole foods? To put it simply, the Atkins diet doesn't put a cap on how much protein you can take in in a day. With keto, you have to mind your macronutrients and keep them in a very specific balance. Without this balance, the liver is not producing ketones for your body, which is what turns you into that fat-burning powerhouse. Too much protein kicks your body out of ketosis, and we'll go into exactly how much protein you should be eating.

How it Works:

As previously stated, the purpose of the ketogenic diet is to put you into ketosis and keep you there. Let's delve a little bit more into the specifics of this principle and what the alternatives are. As we said before, your body can run on either fat or carbs to create energy. What are the differences and benefits of each?

When your body is running on carbohydrates, it metabolizes those into sugar. The sugar is then processed throughout your system to keep you going, and the liver produces insulin so your body can absorb and make use of those sugars. This is the process that gives your body the energy to get through your day.

Now, the problem with running on sugar is that your blood sugar is prone to spiking. This means you have a good burst of energy right after consumption, and a few hours later you feel like you're going to fall asleep on your keyboard. Spikes and crashes are not conducive to a productive, high-energy day. The other problem with spikes is that, once you crash, your system will tell you that you need to put more carbs and sugar in your body, so you feel better. This is because these are the sources your body knows as the most quick and effective way to get out of the slump. This is where we get the urge to snack on things we shouldn't be eating throughout the day, we want to eat late at night because our bodies think we need a little something extra, and it's all one big recipe for excess weight gain.

Now, let's flip the script and take a look at a body that is running on little to no carbs, with a high intake of high-quality fats. Using all the fat in your body, the liver produces ketones. These are then dispersed throughout the body and used to keep you going. Ketones can be regarded as a "clean fuel source," for your body. They keep your energy levels sustainable, keep you feeling better, and keep the fat burning in your body, even when you're completely at rest.

Being on a ketogenic diet means that your body is constantly creating ketones for your body and your brain to use. This means that you're running at peak levels, thinking more clearly, and burning fat like you've never done before. With fat being burned so efficiently and so constantly, your body has no other option than to utilize your excess weight and burn it off at a rate like never before.

You'll lose excess weight, stay satisfied for longer, control your blood sugar with not crashes throughout the day, and you'll give your body a stronger chance at fighting and reversing a laundry list of illnesses that can develop as a result of obesity or poor eating habits. 50% of Americans are projected to develop type 2 diabetes within their lifetime at this stage of society. The problem with a diet that causes your body to burn primarily sugar, is that is doesn't burn the fat, which is being stored in the body.

Insulin tells your body to store fat, so it has something to live on, in the event that food becomes scarce. This is believed to be a holdover from that era we mentioned before, that was prior to modern farming. The thing about today's world is that food is readily accessible to the common American and those periods of starvation never come, so your excess fat goes stored and unused for a period of years.

As previously mentioned, there is a specific balance you need to keep amongst your macronutrients, in order to keep your body in ketosis. Let's examine what the ideal type of daily intake would look like:

- Fat should make up 40% - 70% of your daily calories
- Protein should make up 15% - 30% of your daily calories
- Carbohydrates should make up 5% - 15% of your daily calories and <u>should not exceed 30 grams</u>.
- The results that have been mentioned in this book as regards fat burning and weight loss are all estimated before exercise is factored into the equation. With exercise, your body will be burning even more fat than it would on a regular basis with keto, and you'll have the energy to exercise without feeling exhausted at the end of it. It is not necessary to exercise while on keto, but it certainly helps your cause!

Unlike some other, more drastic diets that are common amongst frequent dieters, keto is one that you can do for life. There are no ill effects to utilizing a keto diet for an indefinite period, and those who have committed to eating in this way as their lifestyle, have found it to be nearly effortless and have found the benefits to be numerous.

In the next chapter, we'll list some recipes for you to try when getting yourself all set to live the keto life!

Chapter 2: Your Quick Keto Recipes

A major roadblock in committing to and getting started on a new regimen is finding foods that you like. If you're eating food that is bland or not to your liking, your chances of staying committed to that regimen are far lower. Another problem that can make it difficult to stick to a healthier regimen is that you don't feel as full after you've eaten some of the approved foods for that regimen.

Putting together a meal plan that is made up of recipes you like, foods that satisfy you, and flavors that excite your palate is a very effective tool for longevity. We've put together 10 recipes that span breakfast, lunch, and dinner so you can get started on the regimen that will help you to achieve your goals.

There are some dietary staples you should know about when it comes to keto. These are things you should keep in your cupboard at all times.

- Coconut oil – you will find this to be incredibly useful to you in your cooking. It has plenty of healthy fats in it and it's packed with nutrients your body needs.
- Erythritol or Monk Fruit Sugar – these are all-natural, sugar-free, calorie-free sweeteners. Lessening your dependency on sweeteners is definitely a great direction

to go in, but for the times when you need some sweetness, these are two great options.

- MCT oil – MCT stands for Multi-Chain Triglycerides, which help your body boost ketone production. You can use it in your bulletproof coffee, which is explained in this chapter. While it is derived from coconut oil, it is flavorless. This is a bonus if you're not a fan of coconut flavor but would still like the many benefits they offer.

- Coconut flour – this does carry the flavor and smell of coconut but holds up very well to being used in the same ways that you would use a grain flour. It's perfect for baking, thickening, and other uses in which flour would come in handy.

- Keto-friendly snacks – this includes things like nuts and beef jerky. Find snacks that fit your day, which you can use to fill in the gaps when and where you need to, so you don't go hungry. Finding the right balance in what you need to eat each day can take some time, so don't be afraid to have a snack here or there that fits into your macros.

- Condiments that don't naturally contain sugar – these are essential to adding flavor and moisture to dishes, so don't shy away from things like mustard or mayonnaise if they fit in with your daily macros.

- Spices – Flavor is the answer to loving the foods you cook at home! Learn what spices, herbs, and seasonings you like and keep them in your kitchen *always*!

Bulletproof Coffee

Total prep time & cooking time: 5 min.

Yields: 1 serving

Ingredients:

1 c. coffee, freshly brewed

2 tbsp. unsalted butter

1 tbsp. MCT oil or coconut oil

Instructions:

1. Brew your coffee to your liking.
2. Combine butter, oil, and coffee into the blender and mix until smooth and frothy.
3. Serve and enjoy!

Scrambled Eggs with Avocado

Total prep time & cooking time: 10-15 min.

Yields: 1 serving

Ingredients:

3 eggs

½ avocado

Salt

Pepper

Garlic powder

Instructions:

1. In a medium bowl, whisk eggs with salt and garlic powder to taste. Beat until the seasonings are evenly incorporated.
2. In a medium skillet or frypan, add oil or butter to keep eggs from sticking, then pour the egg mixture once the pan is hot.
3. Using a spatula, keep the eggs moving in the pan as they cook, so an even cook is achieved throughout the eggs.
4. Slice avocado to preference and arrange on a plate, then plate your scrambled eggs.
5. OPTIONAL: Top with a little bit of black pepper or hot sauce for extra flavor

Breakfast Casserole

Total prep time & cooking time: 10-15 min.

Yields: 12 servings

Ingredients:

1 lb. pork breakfast sausage (loose, not links)

½ c. yellow onion, diced.

2 c. zucchini, diced

2 c. green cabbage, finely shredded

3 large eggs

½ c. mayonnaise

2 tsp. yellow mustard

1 tsp. ground sage

1 ½ c. shredded cheddar cheese

Cayenne pepper to taste

Instructions:

1. Preheat oven to 375° F.
2. In a large frypan, cook pork sausage until mostly browned.
3. Add onion, zucchini, and cabbage to frypan and continue to cook until completely browned.

4. In a large mixing bowl, combine eggs, mayonnaise, mustard, sage, 1 cup of cheddar cheese, and add cayenne, salt, and pepper to taste. Mix well until thoroughly combined.

5. In an oiled baking dish, layer ingredients from frypan, topping with egg mixture. In a large salad bowl, layer lettuce and top with cheese, bacon, tomatoes, egg, and dressing of your choice. Mix well and enjoy!

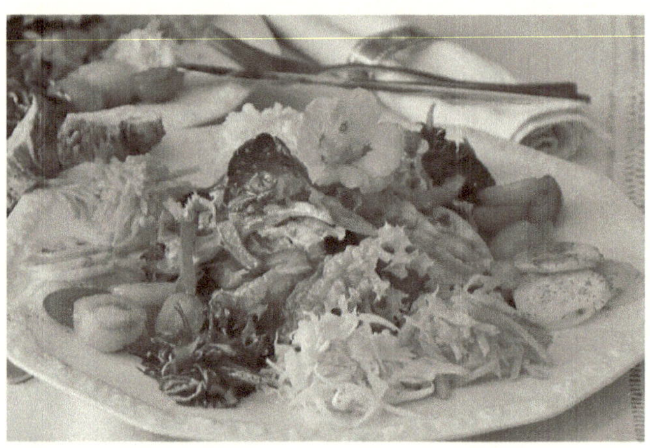

(Cobb Salad)

Sesame Beef Coleslaw

Total prep time & cooking time: 20-25 min.

Yields: 4 servings

Ingredients:

1 lb. ground beef

1 c. coleslaw mix

2 tsp. soy sauce

2 tsp. sriracha

1 tsp. rice wine vinegar

1 ½ tsp. sesame oil

2 tbsp. sesame seeds

Instructions:

1. In a medium frypan, combine all ingredients and mix well. Cook until meat is fully browned.
2. Top with sesame seeds and mix until well combined.
3. Serve and enjoy!

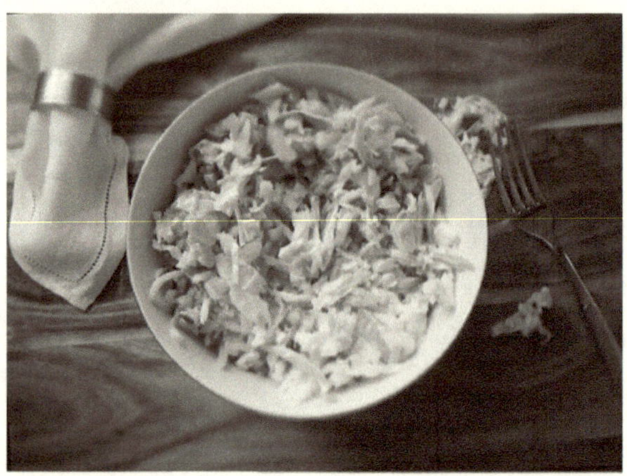

(Beef Coleslaw)

Steamed Chicken with a Asian Twist

Total prep time & cooking time: 20-25 min.

Yields: 1 serving

Ingredients:

1 thinly cut or pounded-out chicken breast

1 bulb bok choy, cleaned

1 tsp. ginger, minced

1 tbsp. fresh basil, sliced

½ tbsp. sesame oil

Instructions:

1. On your cutting board, give your chicken a light coating of salt and pepper to taste, on one side. It's a thin cut, do you don't want to overpower it with pepper.
2. In your steamer, place chicken for about five minutes per side. When you flip the chicken, add bok choy into the steamer and cover until finished.

3. Slice chicken into even pieces, top with ginger basil mixture, plate with book choy and serve!

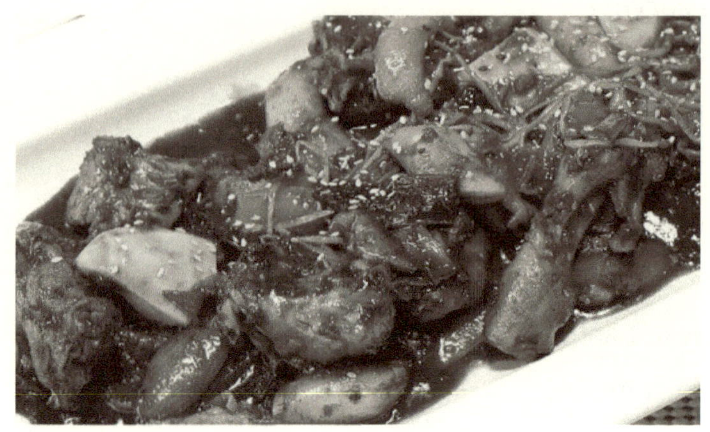

(Steamed chicken)

Baked Paprika Chicken

Total prep time & cooking time: 20-25 min.

Yields: 4 servings

Ingredients:

1 lbs. chicken breasts

2 lemons, quartered

¼ c. olive oil

2 cloves garlic, minced

1 tsp. ground black pepper

1 tsp. smoked paprika

1 tsp. kosher salt

2 tsp. hot paprika

1 tsp. oregano

Instructions:

1. Preheat oven to 425° F.
2. In a small bowl, combine all ingredients except chicken breasts and lemons and mix thoroughly.

3. With a brush or spoon, coat the chicken breasts in the spice mixture and bake for 20 minutes, or until an internal temperature of 165° F is achieved.

4. Squeeze lemon juice over chicken and serve!

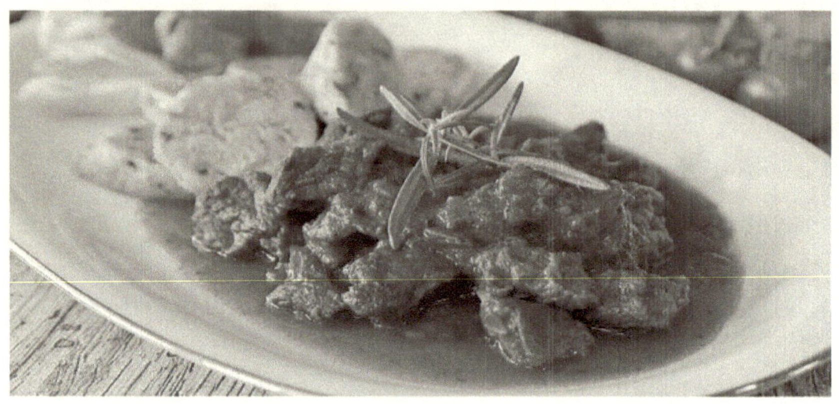

(Paprika Chicken)

Lettuce Tacos

Total prep time & cooking time: 20-25 min.

Yields: 4 servings

Ingredients:

1 lb. ground beef

1 head iceberg or butter lettuce

1 tomato, diced

1 c. sour cream

1 c. shredded cheddar cheese

½ tsp pepper

½ tsp salt

1 ½ tsp cumin

½ tsp paprika

½ tsp onion powder

½ tsp garlic powder

¼ tsp chili powder

Instructions:

1. In a small bowl, mix all your seasonings and set aside.
2. Cut as many leaves of lettuce as you will need for taco shells, rinse well, and pat   dry.
3. Dice tomatoes to your preference. These will be used to top your tacos.
4. Mix half of your seasoning mixture into the meat and work it through, using your hands. You may need to knead it

like dough. Heat butter or olive oil in a medium frypan until it begins to smoke, then add meat. Cook until nearly browned, then add the second half of your seasoning.

5. Mix the seasoning into the meat thoroughly and complete cooking.

6. Spoon taco meat into your lettuce shells, top with cheese, tomatoes, and sour cream to your preference and enjoy!

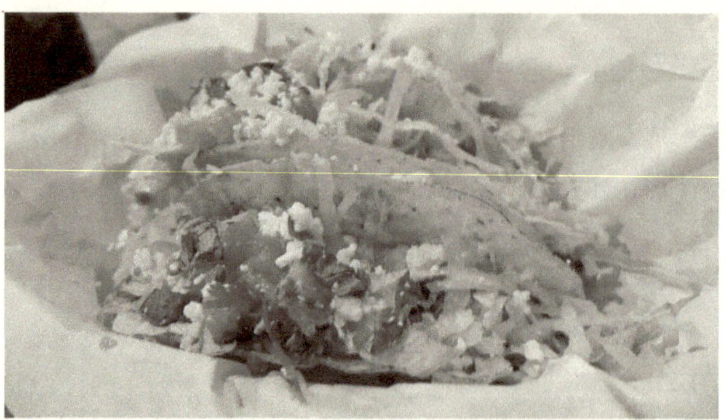

(lettuce Tacos)

Lamb Chop with Feta Salad

Total prep time & cooking time: 20-25 min.

Yields: 1 serving

Ingredients:

2 c. baby leaf spinach, rinsed

1-2 oz. feta cheese

1 6-8 oz. lamb chop

1-2 tbsp. salted butter

1 sprig rosemary

2 cloves garlic, smashed

Salt

Black pepper

Garlic powder

Onion Powder

Instructions:

1. Rinse spinach and set aside to drain any excess water, or spin
    if you have a salad spinner.
2. Lay your lamb chop on a cutting board and give a generous
    sprinkling of each of your seasonings on either side, rubbing
    them in as you do.

3. Heat a medium frypan, ensuring to get the temperature such that the meat will sizzle as soon as it touches it. Place the chop in the pan and fry for 2-3 minutes.

4. Place butter in pan just before you're ready to flip, to give it time to melt a little bit.

5. Flip your chop and place the sprig of rosemary and crushed cloves of garlic on top. Tilt the pan so the melted butter pools on one side and, using a spoon, generously pour the melted butter onto the top of the chop several times in rapid succession. This will infuse the meat with the butter and give you juicy, delicious steak.

6. Top your salad greens with the feta, a drizzle of olive oil, and salt and pepper to taste.

7. Mix salad, plate, and serve!

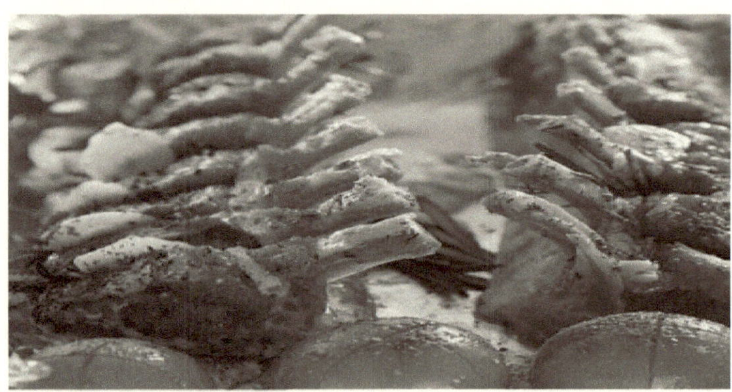

(Lamb Chops)

Buttery Steak & Broccoli

Total prep time & cooking time: 20-25 min.

Yields: 1 serving

Ingredients:

1 head broccoli

1 6-8 oz. steak (your choice of cut)

1-2 tbsp. salted butter

1 sprig rosemary

Salt

Black pepper

Garlic powder

Onion powder

Instructions:

1. Cut the florets from the head of broccoli and rinse them thoroughly.
2. Lay your steak on a cutting board and give a generous sprinkling of each of your seasonings on either side, rubbing them in as you do.
3. Once rinsed, steam the broccoli until a bright, vibrant green color forms on the floret stems and you can stick a fork through it.

4. Heat a medium frypan, ensuring to get the temperature
    such that the meat will sizzle as soon as it touches it.
    Place the steak in the pan and fry for 2-3 minutes.

5. Place butter in pan just before you're ready to flip, to give
    it time to melt a little bit.

6. Flip your steak and place the sprig of rosemary on top.
    Tilt the pan so the melted butter pools on one side and,
    using a spoon, generously pour the melted butter onto
    the top of the steak several times in rapid succession. This
    will infuse the meat with the butter and give you juicy,
    delicious steak.

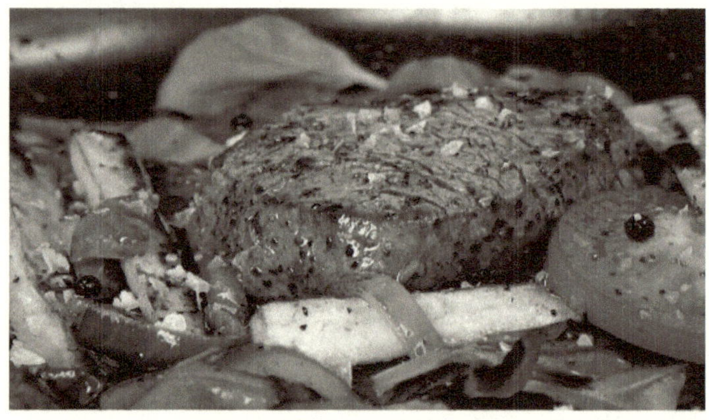

(Steak and vegetables)

Chapter 3: What are the Most Common Mistakes?

Eliminating the "if only Ii had known," moments is a great step toward success in any regimen. In this chapter, we'll discuss some of the most common issues, misconceptions, and mistakes one can make when trying to do a ketogenic diet. Let the experience of many others guide you toward doing what is right for you and your regimen!

<u>Forgetting the Moderate-Protein Part</u>

Possibly the most common error that people make while doing a ketogenic diet is plummeting the carbohydrate intake, without making any adjustments to the amount of fat or protein being taken in. As we've explored previously, having too much protein in your diet can kick you out of ketosis. Having too little of the high-quality fats we need will do the same.

Remember that you are re-training your body to use fat as its primary fuel source. If you're not putting enough of the right kinds of fats into your diet, then you're not going to have the success you would otherwise. You want to ensure that you are keeping your fat intake at 40%-70% of your daily calories. It is best to get this number as close to 70% as possible, and to make sure that the foods that contain those fats, also contain things your body can use, like Omega-3 fatty acids.

The reason it's best to keep your protein within that 15% - 30% range is because your body will take that excess protein and metabolize it into sugar. This puts your body back into that same mode it was in, using sugar as its fuel source. Now, if you go down this road and you continue with a protein intake above 30% per day, your body is using that excess protein, but it's not using excess fat. You're no longer burning your excess fat and additionally, you're not going to feel as energetic, because that protein isn't enough to keep you running all day long.

This will start you on a slippery slope toward feeling hungry or unsatisfied, snacking more, adding more carbohydrates, etc., until you're forced to give up "keto," because it wasn't working. This is not how all scenarios work, but it is common enough that you should be made aware of the possibility.

If it's possible, limit your protein to about 20% a day, so you're on the lower end of that range, and your body will use all the fat you're eating and the excess fat you may have in your body. If you feel that 20% is too low, like you don't have enough energy, or like something might be wrong, consult with your physician about how tweaks can be made to your daily intake, so you feel your absolute best.

Remember, keto is a low-carb, high-fat, *moderate-protein* diet. Never forget that last bit!

Eating Hidden Carbs

As we've explained, it is best to keep your carbohydrate consumption as low as possible. This means that of your daily food intake, no more than 5% - 15% should be carbohydrates. A good rule to go by is no more than 30 grams of carbohydrates per day. This is a very low number for carbohydrates, which is why it's so important to keep your eye on it.

Eating healthy can mean finding snacks and foods that are specifically marketed for the diet or regimen you're doing. The pitfall is that they may say something like, "fat-free," but still contain 36 grams of sugar. The way to avoid the problems that come from situations such as these, is to look at the Nutritional Facts label on the side of the packaging.

Be aware of what the serving sizes are, how much of each of your macros will be coming from that serving, and if it will be filling enough to warrant the number of carbohydrates in it. For instance, you could feasibly eat a potato, but the carbohydrates are so high, that you would be unable to eat any others throughout the day. This limits your nuts, some of your vegetables, and even some meats. Knowing what you're eating is such an important part of living a healthier lifestyle.

Some vegetables have more carbohydrates than you might think, so it's a good idea to look at the nutritional facts, which are listed online or in calorie tracking apps. Using your smartphone as a tool in your weight loss is a great way to ensure you're not tripping yourself up by eating carbs that are hidden from view. Here are some foods you might not have expected to have carbohydrates:

- Onion – 10g of carbohydrates in one medium onion
- Corn – 31.5g in one cup
- Beet – 17g in one cup
- Sweet Potato – 26.2g in one medium potato
- Raisins – 34g in 1.5 ounces
- Beans – 20g in one cup
- Orange – 15.4g in one medium orange
- Chickpeas – 128g in one cup
- Apple – 25g in one medium apple
- Grapefruit – 10g in one medium grapefruit
- Mango – 25g in one cup
- Dates – 18g in one date
- Pear – 27g in one medium pear
- Yogurt – 11.4g in one cup of plain yogurt
- Lentils – 40g in one cup
- Honey – 17.3g in one tablespoon
- Blueberries – 21.4g in one cup
- Peas – 30g in one cup
- Cashews – 8g in one ounce
- Pistachios – 8g in one ounce

Fruit in general can be a tricky food group to navigate when you're working on keeping to a low-carb regimen. However, you'll find that the best fruits for a low-carb diet are berries and honeydew melon.

We also mentioned above, that nuts are a common snack option on a low-carb regimen, but you will find that some have a higher carbohydrate count than others. With nuts, you'll find that pecans, Brazil nuts, and macadamia nuts are the best-suited ones for this type of diet.

Lack of Portion Control

Some people are diving headlong into a ketogenic diet with this notion that, as long as a food has little to no carbohydrates in it, there is no need to monitor or limit the intake. Portion control is part and parcel to any diet, no matter how restrictive it is. Always remember that the key to weight gain is *excess*.

It's true that your main focus should be on the overall intake and the percentages of your macronutrients in that intake. This doesn't mean that you'll be able to lose weight while eating 6,000 calories per day. At that point, your body is taking on more than it can feasibly use in one single day, and you don't want to overload yourself.

Using a calorie-tracking app, or just keeping a food journal with your macros in it, is a great way to get an accurate picture of what your portions should look like. You don't have to commit to logging your calories each day, if that's not something you like doing, or if you don't find it helpful. But using it for a metric at the beginning to give you a better idea of what you're taking in is *strongly* advised.

Not Getting Enough Fat

Not getting enough of the fat you need to help your body run can make it difficult to get through your day without feeling too hungry, or like you need to snack. Remember that fat is the primary source of energy that your body is trying to use. You can't run off of fat if you're not putting any in your system.

Think of the fat that you put into your body like putting gasoline in a car. If you run out of gas, your car won't go, will it? It has no fuel on which to run and while it may run for a few miles with that needle on E, it will eventually peter out until you put more into your system.

Don't neglect this part of your diet, and don't forget to keep your intake up to 70% so your body has all it needs. If you're eating enough of the right fats, you'll have more energy than you know what to do with and you'll stay fuller for longer periods of time.

Ensure that you're looking to the right sources for fat, as well. Some foods may not have as much fat as you think, while others may surprise you and have more than you initially thought. Some of the best sources of fat per serving are:

- Eggs
- Fish
- Nuts
- Avocados
- Chia Seeds
- Flaxseeds
- Olive Oil
- Coconut Oil
- Full-Fat Yogurt

Filling up on the Wrong Kinds of Fat

All fats are not created equal and your body cannot produce a lot of energy to run on if the wrong fats are going into your body. If you're getting your fat primarily from red meat, bacon, butter, and cheese, you will notice some drawbacks.

Let's go back to that car metaphor. Your body is like a high-end sports car. In order to run well, your body needs premium fuel. If you're putting regular fuel into the tank, it will run for a while, but you'll find that you'll have some pretty severe engine trouble as time goes on. You need to make sure that you're putting that premium fuel into your tank and keeping your system running like a well-oiled machine.

The best places to get your fat are nuts, olives, fish, avocados, coconut oil, flaxseeds and chia seeds. A little research goes a long way when finding the foods that will do the most good for your body. Find your favorite sources of fat and make sure they become staples of your diet.

Not Measuring Your Macros

Using an app or a journal to measure the fats, protein, and carbs you're taking on each day is the best way to make sure that you're getting the right amounts. If you're not tracking them, you could be getting less fat than you need, or more carbs than you need. Tracking really is the best way to make sure, and it only takes a couple of minutes out of each day to log all that you're eating.

If you've been avoiding logging your food intake, and you've found that you've plateaued, download a calorie-tracking app. From there, do your best to recall what you've eaten in the last three days and log it. Look at the average macros between those three days and see if you can spot any problem areas. If everything looks to be in order, then you may need to look elsewhere for the cause.

If you find a problem area in your intake over those three days, logging your food could help you to make sure you're getting all the fat, carbs, and protein you need without going too far in one direction or another. Ketosis is such an important part of keto; some might say it *is* the diet. Ensure that you're doing everything in your power to get into ketosis and stay there.

Not Measuring Your Ketones

There are ways to measure the ketones that your body is producing. This will tell you how hard your body is working to burn fat in your body and testing those levels frequently will tell you if your ketone production is consistent. If your body isn't producing enough ketones, that could mean that you need to make some adjustments to your diet.

Ensure that you're closely following the guidelines of a keto diet and that you're not taking on too much or too little of the nutrients you need. If it seems that you're eating everything you should be eating, but you're still not seeing the results when testing your ketone levels, you should speak with your physician and get their recommendations for getting you back into ketosis.

All dietary changes should be made with the consultation and advice of your physician.

Too Much Dairy

Dairy is a very common allergen. Lactose intolerance is a very prevalent issue and it can manifest in a wide range of ways. This could mean that you could have an allergy to lactose and not even know it, if you didn't know to look for these symptoms. Keep an eye out for acne, allergies, asthma, congestion, constipation, diarrhea, irritable bowel, post-nasal drip, sinusitis, weight gain, and more.

It is best to eliminate dairy as a main source of fat and protein, as it can come with a host of issues. For clearer skin, better health, and smoother weight loss, keeping dairy to a minimum is the best option. The fats in dairy are an example of the types of fats you should limit or avoid when working to stay in ketosis, to lose weight, and to live a healthy life.

Neglecting Gut Health

If you've been doing a lot of research on diets and why they're important, you may have been reading some things about maintaining good gut health. Maintaining gut health means giving your microbiome everything it needs to thrive, so you can stay at your healthiest. This might sound a little bit nebulous, so let's go into what the microbiome is and why it's important to your health.

The human microbiome refers to the host of microorganisms that live and thrive in your gut. These are the little workers that keep our system running the way that it should and keeping us feeling our best. By giving the microbiome the right things to feed on, we keep those organisms thriving, which helps us avoid health issues and conditions like weight gain, hyperglycemia, high cholesterol, and other issues.

Ensure that the foods you're taking in each day are foods that your microbiome can use to give you good health in return. Some of the best things to eat in order to help with gut health are bone broth that is packed with grass-fed collagen, minerals from supplements, and kimchi. Do some research into other foods you might like that can promote a healthy microbiome and prevent leaky gut.

Leaky gut is a gastrointestinal issue wherein the intestinal wall thins, and nutrients and organisms can "leak" out. Taking on more grass-fed collagen can contribute to a thicker, healthier intestinal wall that keeps everything in its place. Bone broth can be made at home, or you can buy the type you need at a health foods store, or in the health foods section of your favorite grocery store.

Not Drinking Enough Water

Many people who are doing a ketogenic diet can find themselves having some problems with constipation, cottonmouth, or aches. These are symptoms of dehydration and could mean that you need to be drinking more water than you currently are. If you're having trouble figuring out how much water you should be drinking, there is a rule of thumb that you can follow.

The best rule to follow when deciding how much water to drink, is to drink 4 ounces of water for ever gram of carbohydrates you're taking on. If you're eating 30g of carbohydrates, this means 120 oz., of water will be needed in your system then. When you're drinking this amount of water, your body will be flushing everything through in the way that it should be, and you won't find yourself feeling constipated or dehydrated any longer.

Why is water consumption so important when you're doing a low-carb diet? Now that your body isn't taking on carbs, your body's capacity for water retention is much lower than it once was. While this is largely a positive thing, you will need to ensure you're drinking enough water each day to ensure you have enough water in your system at any given time. This also means you need to make sure that you're getting enough electrolytes when you drink, so the water that you do drink ends up going further each time.

Drinking enough water ensures that all the systems in your body, including your gut, are well-lubricated, impurities are being flushed through your system, and all the parts of your tract are running smoothly!

Not Using Salt with Minerals

Iodized table salt has been associated with a host of medical issues, not the least of which is high blood pressure. This is a large part of what a lot of people tend to cut salt out of their diet entirely. The thing about this is that salt is actually an electrolyte that your body needs in order to function properly, so cutting it out entirely can cause some issues in your body.

The best way to keep salt in your diet, and to keep your health on an even keel, is to use salt that has minerals in it. This means using sea salt, Himalayan pink salt, or ancient salt. These are typically rich in minerals that your body can use to hydrate you and to thrive.

Minerals are something that are missed by a lot of dieters who aren't sure which supplements they should be taking. Having minerals in your diet is essential to overall health. Minerals, as well as vitamins, are essential parts of overall health. Consult with your physician about also adding vitamins and minerals to your daily regimen to ensure you're getting all that you need in order to stay healthy!

Chapter 4: Your 5 Golden Rules

<u>Do Not Eat in Front of a Screen</u>

Studies show us that eating in front of the television can open us up for some trouble. It is best to eat at the table, with those in your household. Mealtimes are a great time to open the floor for one-on-one communication, as well! When you think of the dinner table, it can often just be the place where you keep the fruit bowl or the mail. It helps to see it as the round table of your home, where important conversations, catching up, and sharing a meal together all occur.

The first reason to avoid eating in front of the television may strike you as somewhat basic at first. Watching television is a very common toll we use to become distracted. It is entertaining, to be certain, but it also helps us to decompress, unwind, and stop thinking about the events of the day for an hour or two in the evenings. One of the things that comes with this distraction is sort of a disconnection from what's going on in our immediate environments, even if it's something we're actively doing.

So, while you're distracted by what you're watching on television with the fork in your hand, you might be so preoccupied that autopilot takes over, causing you to eat more than you might do otherwise. If you're watching television, taking bite after bite for the duration of the episode or movie, you might find that you've eaten too much, too fast, and you feel bloated or not as full. Being engaged in conversation with others can cause us to put the fork down in between bites, talk a little bit, let the food digest a little bit, go in for the next bite, and so on. This gives the body a much better chance to properly digesting the food you're taking on, as well as allowing you to feel full, with no bloating at the end of your meal.

In addition to eating more than is necessary, eating in front of the television can lead to bloating and digestive issues. This is thanks, in part, to that "autopilot" I mentioned, that can cause you not to chew your food as much as may be needed for proper digestion. Chewing your food helps to break the food down and introduce enzymes that help your food to more easily and properly digest once it enters your digestive system. If you're not chewing properly, you may have some troubles with bloating, diarrhea, constipation, or the speed of your metabolism. Chewing your food is very important and spacing out the bites as mentioned in the previous paragraph, are great ways to ensure that your body can properly use the food you work hard to give it!

Depending on what you're watching, you might find that you come across food commercials. Food commercials are specifically designed to make you feel hungry, so you go out and buy that burger, pizza, taco, pasta, etc. If you're working hard on eating only the healthiest foods, you might split the difference, wander into the kitchen, and grab a little something extra since you were just eating dinner, it didn't quite fill you up, and now you just need a little something extra. While that trip to the kitchen *is* an extra step and thus an extra deterrent in getting more food, watching television while eating will only make you feel like you need to eat more than you really do.

Say you have some junk food saved in the cabinet for a rainy day, you eat your dinner in front of the television, see a commercial for something that is terrible for you. It looks so enticing, you think, well I do have those snacks in the kitchen. Bringing those snacks back to the couch is a recipe for overeating, lack of satisfaction, and no snacks for later. Save your snacks, eat at the table!

It's no secret that watching television has some rather addictive properties to it. In fact, we have given the name "binge" to watching a lot of a particular show all at once. It is addictive and like with many things, taking it in on a large scale can lead to problems. Part of the addictive nature of television is that you can form other habits while watching television without even realizing it. If you're eating in front of the television every time you watch, it's going to become nearly impossible to watch television without feeling the need to eat *something*.

This can make it hard to watch your favorite movies or shows in between mealtimes without feeling hungry! Diets and lifestyle changes are hard enough without these subconscious and subliminal triggers coming in to sabotage us! Because of this, it's best to take a proactive approach to things and ensure that you're able to get the entertainment you want and deserve, without this level of added difficulty.

So, what is the best way in which to reset this cycle of behavior? When changing a habit, it's best to start with a clear intention for what the new habit should be. Saying, "I'm not going to eat in front of the television," with no decision on what you *will* do instead, leaves you open to making decisions that might be contrary to progress while you're in the moment. So, what should your new habit in front of the television be? Should it be to sit there quietly and enjoy the entertainment? Should it be something more proactive than that?

A creative tool that some have found to be largely effective is taking up a hobby that involves both hands. Doing something like crochet, drawing, coloring, or painting while watching television has been proven to keep the mind more engaged and preoccupied. In these cases, thinking about food doesn't happen nearly as often as it may have done previously before the hobby was used in this way.

What is something fun and engaging that you can do while watching television to keep cravings at bay? Think of a few and see how those serve you! We do have a suggestion for something engaging and proactive you can do while watching television, and that's the next item in this chapter.

Exercise While You're Watching

Television

Getting started on a workout regimen that can assist you in your weight loss can be really difficult, especially if you've never done such a thing in the past. When you first get into doing workouts, the first place that a lot of people like to go is cardio. Doing workouts that get your heart pumping, your blood moving, and your sweat dripping, are a great way to go. This means things like the elliptical, a stationary bike, the treadmill, arc trainers, etc.

Now, when you're working to push yourself through the huffing, puffing, and burning, it can be rough. If your whole thought process is taken up by the huffing, puffing, and burning, it could seemingly take forever to get through any of it. A lot of people are familiar with using music as a way to put your focus on something familiar, a rhythm to follow, and to stimulate the pleasure centers of your brain.

The principle behind watching television during a workout is more of less the same, while having another principle behind it as well. Those of us who are into watching television as part of our daily or nightly routine, are subject to packing on a couple extra pounds here and there, because it's a largely sedentary activity aside from the occasional laundry-folding or crafting project that we might do from time to time.

Using television as a way to distract ourselves through a workout in the evenings could be a great start. This is a way to get some activity into that time in our evenings. It's also a great way to feel a little less guilty about watching seven episodes of a show in one sitting. On top of this, you'll find that working out before bedtime will help you to feel even more rested than you already would with the benefits of keto on your side.

When distracting yourself through a workout, you will notice some benefits that will help you in your path toward a more vigorous regimen. For one thing, it's pretty hard to believe someone who says that they enjoy their exercise routine. If you're not used to physical activity, it can feel horrible and you might think people who say they enjoy it are either lying to your face or are certifiably insane. The first key (of many) in making a workout regimen into something you can actually enjoy, is to pair it with something that you currently enjoy.

As mentioned previously, music can be one of these enjoyable things that distracts you, puts you into a better mindset to achieve what you want to achieve with your workout, and can get you though it. Television has these same benefits, as well as some others. The principle behind keeping yourself distracted through your workout is that it is a dissociative strategy, as opposed to an associative strategy. Let's go into what this means in basic terms.

An associative strategy means that you're looking within. You're focused on the body, what it's feeling, what it's doing, how the workout is going, and your thoughts that relate specifically to your body and the effects on it. The benefit of being in an associative mindset when working out is that you can feel when you're pushing too hard, or you can know immediately if you're able to push a little harder and get better results from your workout. Those who are entirely focused within tend to notice a mental clarity and a lack of stressful thought processes about the day behind or ahead of them, problems in life, or other things that might otherwise cause us to shy away from our workout. Your mind homes in on your workout, your body, and the activities at hand.

Being completely unfocused on those other parts of your life, working on getting your body moving, and focusing on that effort you're putting out can be helpful in other ways as well.

Many who use this method of working out find that, once they complete their workout and resume other daily activities, they have more clarity on subjects or situations that had been causing them some difficulty before the workout. It helps to take a step back from the situations, give your mind a break, refresh, and look at it all again with a fresh set of eyes, so to speak.

Alternatively, a dissociative strategy is one that takes your mind off of your body and what it's doing. This approach has a wider range of what you could be focused on, because daydreaming and thinking about other things is still considered dissociative. You're not focused on your body and what it's doing right in that moment. This could mean being focused on the music you're listening to, what you're going to make for dinner, the conversation you had with a friend the other day, or the show that's currently on the television in front of you. The benefits of this approach are different than the associative approach, but they're not necessarily better or worse in any way. They can, however, be more useful at different stages of your workout regimen. We'll discuss why later on in this section.

The dissociative approach is the one that allows you step back from that huffing, puffing, and burning we mentioned previously. Removing those from your primary focus can sort of pave the way for a more positive thought process or a better overall mindset while you're working out. At the beginning of a regimen such as this, it offers a sort of reprieve to your mind to find enjoyment in the process of watching television while going through the workout. This will help to ease you into that transition.

Once you start to get into the rhythm of working out during your television time, you could find that some positive changes come about as a result. You might find that doing this resets the addictive response that can often accompany television time, which is the compulsion to eat. If you're busy working out, you're less likely to feel the need to snack in front of the television. Due to the addictive quality of television, you could also find that your attraction to television time is lessened, thus minimizing your viewing time, or you could find that you form a sort of addiction to the endorphins you generate while watching television. There are worse addictions than fitness, right?

Now, as you continue your workouts and you find that you can do more arduous things in the time you have, you might find the distraction of television makes it more difficult to achieve the goals you want to achieve. This is the point at which you might find that it's best to switch the medium of distraction to something like music, podcasts, talk radio, audio books or the like. If you find that those methods are too distracting, you might find that the associative strategy mentioned previously is the best method for you to get through your workout with the best results!

If you're interested in using your viewing time as workout time, there are a few ways in which you could go about it. Using the things on the television as cues can help you to switch up the thing you're doing and act as your stopwatch. It has been said that you never truly know how long a minute is until you have to run for sixty seconds straight. Television might be the ticket to making that sixty seconds tick by before you know it. Once you get past that first minute, you'll surprise yourself and, before too long, twenty minutes will breeze right by you. Take a look at the next few suggestions and see if there is a regimen here that you feel you could use to help you get started!

Basic Cardio

Watch one episode of your show and do cardio (running, walking, elliptical, treadmill, etc.) for one full episode, one and a half if you're watching without commercials.

If you're binge-watching something on a streaming service, do cardio for two episodes (or 40-ish minutes) and take a rest for one. If you're up to it, hop back on for the next two.

Body Weight (with commercials)

At each commercial break, stop the exercise you're doing and shift to the next!

Sit-ups

Jumping jacks

Lunges

Chair dips

Squats

Hip raises

Body Weight (without commercials)

While you're watching your shows or movie, set a stopwatch to go off every five minutes or so and do the following exercises for five minutes each.

Sit-ups

Jumping jacks

Lunges

Chair dips

Squats

Hip raises

As time goes on, you can mix and mingle exercises with cardio as works best for you. As you begin to work extra things in, you could do:

Cardio for one episode

Sit-ups for five minutes

Jumping jacks for five minutes

Lunges for five minutes

Chair dips for five minutes

Cardio for another episode

Squats for five minutes

Hip raises for five minutes

Planks for two minutes on each side (alternate each minute if necessary)

Rest for five minutes

Cardio for one episode.

Every instance where "episode" is used as a unit of measurement, this refers to 20-minute episodes. Episodes that are closer to 40 or 50 minutes should be broken up differently, so make sure to pay attention to that.

Snack Mostly on Fruits and Vegetables

There are a lot of reasons that you may feel like you need snacks in between meals. Eating one snack between each mealtime is a great way to keep you going, but you might find that you're feeling like having more than that. In the event that you feel the need to snack, having cut and prepared vegetables on hand to eat is a great way to keep yourself in check and to make sure you're not snacking on foods that aren't conducive to your goals. Let's take a look at some of the reasons why we might feel compelled to snack a little bit more than we probably should.

Not Eating Enough at Mealtimes or Not Enough of the Right Nutrients

If you're not getting enough food in your meals to keep you satisfied, it stands to reason that every time you see a snack, you're going to want it. It also stands to reason that you'll find yourself getting hungry between meals, whether you're looking at food or not. It's important to make sure that the food you're eating has enough in it to keep you satisfied until your next mealtime or scheduled snack.

If you're not certain how much you will need to eat to stay full, run a trial by error. Add more and more vegetables to your meals each time until you've reached a balance that makes you feel full without bloating or pain, but keeps you moving until your next meal. If you find that adding more vegetables doesn't keep you full, consider adding more fat from healthier sources, while keeping an eye on the amount of protein you're taking in.

If you find that you have difficulty staying fed while keeping your macros where they need to be, consider seeing your physician to seek out recommendations on how you can go longer without getting hungry. This is an atypical occurrence when on keto, but it is important to know there is always help and there are always resources to help you get over whatever hurdles you may have.

Too Many Simple Carbohydrates

If you've stepped out of the guidelines of what carbohydrates you're allowed to have on this regimen, you might find that attempts to get back on track are a little harder. You'll feel a little bit hungrier between meals than you would otherwise. If you happen to stray a little bit from the regimen one day and take on more simple carbohydrates than you should, be prepared for a bit more hunger the next day, than you might typically expect.

It is best to ensure you eat a lot of fresh vegetables and healthy fats on that following day. This way, you can stay ahead of the curve and you'll have a better chance of keeping yourself full between your meals.

Dehydration

Believe it or not, your body can mistake dehydration and hunger. As mentioned previously, your body is less able to retain moisture with fewer carbohydrates in your body. Since the hunger and thirst responses come from the same portion of the brain, it can seem like you might need to eat something. This could be analogized as your body giving you a vague command like, "you need to ingest something."

That something might be a nutrient-rich meal, or it could be an electrolyte-rich glass of water! Reach for some water first, wait a little while, and see how you feel before committing to snacking between your meals. You might find that you feel more refreshed and less hungry moving forward!

Stress

You may have some familiarity with stress eating, as it's far from an uncommon occurrence for people who are frequently stressed. One of the many unfortunate things about stress eating is that it doesn't tend to occur in instances of short-term stress. Once someone has been experiencing stress on a semi-frequent basis or more, the body has physical responses that lead to our feeling like we need to eat more. Yet another unfortunate fact of this is that eating under stress can tend to cause excess weight-gain as well.

When you're stressed, there is an elevated production of the hormone cortisol in your body. This is a hormone that can cause motivation for a lot of things, eating included. If you stay stressed, that cortisol continues to course through and cause that response. There are some more aspects to that stress-hunger relationship that are at work as well.

Many studies conducted around stress eating revealed that when participants were experiencing more stress, the foods they reached for were typically higher in sugar, fat, or both. This is an added obstacle that works against you when you're trying to maintain a healthy eating regimen under stress.

Reducing stress could go a long way toward helping you to live a more peaceful, restful, and satisfied life! Here are some methods of stress relief you may be able to use to help you limit the stress you feel from day to day. Look through them and see if there are any that would work for you, which you could work into your daily routine.

Aromatherapy – Strong-smelling candles, oils, and sprays can interact cause your body to produce fewer stress hormones. Consider what aromas are pleasant to you and think about introducing them into your environment on a regular basis to assist with stress!

Assert Yourself – Studies find that if we allow ourselves to be put into situations we don't want, or which make us uncomfortable, it is a recipe for stress. Learning to assert yourself can help you to fight for outcomes and circumstances that ultimately make your life a little bit easier. By knowing what you want, communicating it respectfully, keeping your voice even, and being willing to be present in an uncomfortable situation, you can assert yourself. Get what you need without feeling bad about it!

Avoid Procrastination – By pushing all our tasks until the last possible moment, we leave ourselves with a high-pressure dash to a deadline. This can create stress, and any relaxation done before that dash to the finish, will usually be less restful. Get the most out of the time you have by working hard from the start, then use the time you have left over to get that restful relaxation that you deserve!

Be Grateful – Concentrating on the things in your life for which you can be thankful, gives you a mindset that is able to find more things for which to be grateful. Take just a little bit of time each day and find things for which you can be grateful. As you go on, this will require less and less effort, and you'll find your mindset to be more focused on those things that make you happy to be here with us.

Chew Sugar-Free Gum – While trying to avoid chemical sweeteners if at all possible, chewing sugar-free gum can occupy you and keep you from developing large amounts of stress hormones. Another helpful benefit is this: if you're chewing gum when stress hits you, you won't clench your jaw and tighten up if you're actively chewing! Jaw clenching can lead to pain, a stiff jaw joint, neck pain, headaches and tooth damage.

Cut Out Things and People That Add Stress – Things in your life that cause you stress aren't worth the effort it takes to keep them there. If there are activities, people, items, situations, in your life that are causing you stress to deal with, figure out how to phase them out as quickly as possible, as your long-term health and your overall well-being depend on it. If it's possible to address and change the things about these things that are stressful, that is also very helpful. Don't, however, allow stress to sit in your life and cause you trouble you don't deserve!

Decompress – Lie back, get comfortable, and apply a hot compress to your neck if you find that to be helpful or relaxing. For ten minutes or so, lie there and concentrate on relaxing the muscles in your face, neck, back, chest, arms, legs, and feet. Feel the tension leave your body and resume the rest of your day as a wet noodle!

Deep Breathing – While taking a five-minute break, take the time to do the following. Sit up straight, close your eyes, and place a hand on your abdomen. Breathe in deeply, taking your time to do so and feeling the breath fill your body. Slowly exhale and feel the air as it leaves your body. Repeat at an even pace for five minutes. The goal here is not to hyperventilate, so ensure you're keeping your breath even! Return to your daily routine after this and feel refreshed!

Exercise – Never underestimate the power of getting active and feeling those endorphins! Working out can actually lower the output of stress hormones, and it can contribute to better, more restful sleep. Getting even ten minutes of cardio into your day where you didn't have it before is a great way to help you to reduce stress.

Get Enough Sleep – To pick up on part of what was said in the point above, getting more sleep that is restful is essential to stress reduction. When you're tired, you're less prepared for the things that come at you during the week. The importance of a good night's sleep cannot be understated.

Get Social Support – Getting through any regimen change or life event is difficult without the help of family and friends. Seeking out companionship, affirmation, and reassurances from those who are closest to you will help you to manage the stress that you're feeling. Take the time to talk with them about things that are stressing you out, as well as about other things you can enjoy. Laughing with friends and family can have a wealth of benefits for your health and well-being.

Hydrate – Ensure that you're getting enough water and electrolytes to keep your body hydrated at all times. You may notice that this has come up in a few different sections now. This should tell you how important it is, for so many reasons, for you to stay hydrated. Drink enough water each day to keep you feeling healthy, vivacious, and stress-free!

Indulge in Creativity and Practice your Art – Having a creative outlet that you can spend time working on is a great way to clear your mind of the stressful things going on around you. Throughout the day, our minds can get cluttered by the things that cause us the most stress. Taking time to practice your art or to work on a creative project of yours, gives you time to focus solely on something you like doing. There isn't much room in your mind for nagging thoughts when you're working on something that brings you happiness.

Intimate Contact with Others – Sometimes a hug, kiss, or cuddle from someone we love is just what the doctor ordered. Intimate physical contact lessens the production or stress hormones and increases the production of happiness hormones. Getting more of this in your day is a great way to minimize the stress you feel over the course of a day.

Journaling – Writing down your thoughts on the day or on some of the other things in this list can help you to gain a helpful perspective on things. Just like talking through things, you can often find solutions to problems, gain a better view of the situation, or just feel like you're getting it out of your head. Taking just 15 minutes or so each evening to jot some things down could do a good deal to help you reduce stress from day to day.

Laugh – *Laughter is the best medicine,* as it turns out, isn't just a cliché. It really can do the body good to laugh frequently. In spending time with your friends and family, it's good to talk about things that make you laugh. Spending time laughing releases hormones that can reduce stress, and if you have things to laugh about throughout your day, things won't seem so rough!

Learn to Say No – Feeling compelled to say yes to everything asked of you can lead to a world of stress that you don't need or want. It can lead to people putting a lot of pressure on you without realizing it, giving you responsibilities that you shouldn't have in the first place, and it can overload and stress you out to an extreme. For someone who feels compelled to say yes to things in order to help others, saying no is *work*. It's not something that will come to you overnight, but start practicing saying no when people ask you things. As time goes on, you will get better at saying no to the things you cannot comfortably do.

Part of saying no means knowing what it means to agree to more than you can handle. Agreeing to overwhelm yourself to do something for someone, when you had the option of saying no, is a terrible feeling. It can lead to so much stress that is unnecessary. Always remember this, there are usually others who can do the favor you are being asked. The fact that that person has to keep looking for someone to do that favor for them, is *not* your responsibility.

Leisure Activities – Doing things that you enjoy can impart a lot of light and happiness in your life. If you're stressed, you tend to reflect on the things in your life that are contributing to that condition. If you have more stressful elements in your life than positive ones, you will find yourself in this position more often than is probably healthy. Take the time to impart activities you enjoy into your life, so you have things to keep you happy and balanced.

Listen to Music – Listening to music, as mentioned in a previous section of this chapter, can serve as a distraction from all the things going on in your life that are causing you stress. If you're feeling particularly stressed, turn on some of your favorite music, lie back, and concentrate on what's playing. Allow your mind to wander and get lost in the music, as this will help to boost happiness hormones and reduce stress hormones!

Look at Happy Photos – With social media being as prevalent as it currently is, funny, happy, or cute pictures are much more common in daily life. There is science to support looking at pictures of cute animals, funny scenarios, or even of people that you love, can help to reduce stress. If you have pictures from a vacation you've taken, a project you're proud to have finished, or something else that brought you happiness, looking at them can help you to de-stress a little bit.

Massage – This is one that I know most of us wish we could go do immediately. Massage is such a pleasant sensation and can help to eliminate serious stress and tension in the body. Like decompressing, it allows you to relax all your muscles, clear your mind, and just enjoy the sensation. Aside from the many health benefits that massage can have, reducing stress is a really useful byproduct of getting semi-regular massages.

Meditation – It's possible that you've tried this method of stress reduction, but if you haven't, it could help you to focus, relax, and reduce stress in your life. There are methods of meditation for different focuses and guided meditation is a great place to start if you're not sure how to do it on your own. Meditation could take as much or as little time as you see fit once you get started, so there is no need to feel committed to any specific amount of time.

Mindfulness – Simply put, mindfulness is a completely present state of mind. Being aware of your body, sensations, your surroundings, the situation around you, and what you're doing there. Mindfulness can help with stress by taking you out of the things that are going on outside your immediate environment that might be causing you stress. When you're being mindful, you're much more able to shift your focus to where you want it to go. You can shift your thoughts away from the things that have been causing you difficulty and onto the things you're trying to accomplish right now.

Play with Animals – Playing with an animal that you love can produce oxytocin in your brain, which reduces the production of cortisol, that stress hormone we mentioned previously. There's just something about snuggling with a fuzzy creature that loves you that seems to make everything better, isn't there? Playing with animals, even if you're less familiar with them, can help with this hormone production, so maybe take a trip to the pet store or the petting zoo for a little pick-me-up.

Practice Positive Self-Talk – Life is hard enough without a steady stream of criticisms coming from within you at all hours of the day. Practicing saying good things about yourself, to yourself, can help change the way you think about and see yourself. It may take some forcing at first, or a little extra effort, but before too long, it will become habit. Having yourself as an ally in the things you want to do in life will make things much easier in the long run.

Progressive Muscle Relaxation – This is a non-pharmacological approach to relaxation that can be used to help you relax your muscles, be relieved of stress or anxiety-inducing thoughts, and reduce stress. It does take a little bit of reading to understand how it works, but there is a wealth of resources on how to do this. It could prove very useful to you in eliminating or reducing the stress in your life. It has been found that Progressive Muscle Relaxation can also be a non-pharmacological method used to help treat things such as sports injuries, insomnia, mental disorders, self-esteem, overall mood, and can even make childbirth less painful.

Reassess Your To-Do Lists – Ensure that you're not putting things on your to-do lists that aren't necessary or that only serve to overwhelm you. If you find that you have some days when you're completely free, but others where you're slammed, you might want to consider redistributing your tasks throughout your day. You may find, when reassessing your to-do lists, that you have items on there that could be delegated to others, done at a later date, or dropped entirely! Be realistic about what you can handle, don't overwhelm yourself, and do your best.

Reduce Caffeine Intake – Prolonged use of caffeine can affect your sleep and can make it easier for you to get agitated by the things in your environment. Cutting down on caffeine can be difficult depending on your current usage, but it is worth it in the long term. It is easier on your adrenal system, digestive system, tooth enamel, nail beds, skin, hair, and sleep quality to consume less caffeinated beverages such as energy drinks and coffee. Feel better in and out with less caffeine!

Sing – Singing, like listening to music, can give you that distraction and stress relief. Added to this there is a certain freeing quality about being able to shout lyrics to favorite jams at the top of your lungs. While you're driving home from work or your lunch break, roll up the windows in your car, pump up the music and let it loose! Singing quietly can also be helpful, so don't be afraid to live for the music.

Spend Time with Family and Friends – This can tie in a bit with getting social support. Spending time with those who mean the most to you and relaxing with them is a great way to charge your batteries, so to speak. Talk with them about anything, laugh with them, play games, sing songs, reminisce, and enjoy their company. This is the stuff of life that makes all the stress worth it, so try not to forget that as you're busy living your best life!

Take a Walk – There is a good deal of science to support taking a walk as a valid form of stress reduction. Taking a walk and a quiet moment to observe the pace of things in the outside world can give you a sense of clarity and serenity. The next time you're feeling like you're under immense pressure and you can't make that deadline, take ten minutes, get up, walk around outside, look at the people, flora, and fauna, and relax. Notice the things going on around you and see the good in the world. See how you feel after that and make it a regular thing if you wish!

Yoga – Yoga is a widely-used method of solving a good number of problems. Due to the amount of stretching it entails, it's good for releasing tension from your muscles, it's good for centering your mind as you're encouraged to focus on your muscles and what they're doing, it can be relaxing once you start to feel the release it provides, and much more. It's hard to go wrong in adding yoga to your regimen, as it can be tailored to any skill level. Doing something as simple as being up on all fours, looking up to the ceiling is a pose that can be done my many. See if a beginner's class is available for you and you might find that it's something that could help you!

Pick a couple of these and take steps to implement them in your daily life. Take note of how you feel in general before starting them and keep track as you go. You might be surprised to find that eliminating stress from your life is helping you to achieve more of your goals. Whether those goals have to do only with weight loss or if there's more to it, having less stress will only take you in the right direction toward achieving those goals! Stress can do so much more damage than we may realize; eliminate stress from your life and see what surprising changes come about for you.

Not Eating Mindfully

As mentioned in the stress portion in the snacking section, mindfulness is a mindset that puts you completely in the current moment. You're completely aware of the moment, yourself, your body, sensations and everything that is present with you. When you eat in this type of mindset, you'll be more aware of the food you're putting into your body. There is more to it, but that is the nutshell of mindful eating.

Let's look at what exactly changes when you eat mindfully, as opposed to eating with distractions. When you're eating mindful, you will taste every bite of the food you eat. You're more likely to end your meal feeling satisfied if you take the time to savor the flavors and textures that are in it. Concentrate on how much there is, how much you're taking in each bite, how much chewing you're doing, how it feels to swallow it, and how full you feel.

When you concentrate on these things, you'll remember that you've eaten, you'll feel more satisfied, you'll feel fuller, you'll enjoy your food a bit more, and you won't eat your food so quickly that you inhibit digestion. Chewing your food properly and eating at a slow, even pace is a great way to keep you from eating more than you should or from feeling bloated, over-full, or even still hungry at the end of your meal.

Give this a try and see what changes it makes to the amount of snacking you feel you need to do. When you don't need to snack as much, you will find that you can make your meals mean a little bit more and improve their staying power with lots of healthy fats and a good amount of protein to keep you moving.

Not Enough Sleep

This is one of the things you'll notice being mentioned frequently throughout these sections. Getting insufficient sleep to get you through your day can do so much to set you back. Getting consistently insufficient sleep can have even worse effects that can cause life to seem a little bit bleak. Studies show that lack of sleep can affect many aspects of your life, including depression.

If you find that you're not getting restful sleep, the need to eat or snack could come about as a result. Increased stress, lack of alertness, higher risk for accidents, lowered immune response, clouded thought process, weight gain, and skin conditions are all part of the troubles that can come from getting too little sleep for too long. If you have difficulty getting to sleep, staying asleep, and feeling rested after sleeping, you may want to look into some things you can do to improve things. Getting better sleep and feeling better as a result could take some time, but it's well worth the effort you'll put into it.

Developing and sticking to a steady routine is a great way for your body to know when it's time to sleep. Sleeping at the same time (or thereabouts) each evening will help your body get acclimated and ready to wind down at around the same time each day. Obviously, there will be nights when getting to sleep at a reasonable hour just isn't feasible, but one or two nights here or there shouldn't disrupt your whole regimen. Make a commitment to get back on track as quickly as possible after each deviance, and you'll settle right back into your routine with no issue.

Staying active during the day is a great way to make sure you're nice and ready for bed in the evening. When we stay sedentary throughout the day, you'll find that you have some pent-up energy at the end of it all. Being active in the earlier part of the day will help you in so many ways, sleep being a pretty important one.

Limiting your usage of things like cigarettes and alcohol is a great way of helping you to achieve a more restful sleep. Studies have found that both of these vices can lead to a stimulating effect once their initial effects wear off. While both have been known to have calming or even soothing effects when first used, as they leave the system, it can leave you with a restlessness that can make it difficult to achieve a fully restful sleep.

If you find that you regularly make use of things like cigarettes and alcohol, cutting back your usage could be beneficial for your overall health. Both vices contribute to heart disease, cancer, high blood pressure, and many more illnesses that could significantly reduce quality of life in chronic users. Quitting these things could help you to see even more results from your keto regimen than you may have been able to otherwise.

It is recommended to cease consumption of media on electronic devices for at least 30 minutes before going to bed. Doing so allows your brain to acclimate to the lack of stimulation that those types of devices provide. If you're using these devices right up until or even while you're in bed, you might find that the rest you're getting isn't as restful as it could be. Try reading quietly, doing a puzzle, or even meditating before heading to bed and see what kind of improvements you notice in the length and quality of your sleep.

Ambient light is found to disrupt the production of melatonin in your brain. Your brain thinks these lights are present because you should be paying attention to them, so it will hold back that hormone. If you do your best to eliminate light before bedtime, as well as to sleep in a room that is as close to pitch black as possible, your brain will produce the melatonin you need to get off to sleep with fewer issues. Staying asleep when your brain is producing melatonin at a higher rate is easier as well.

A study conducted by the National Sleep Foundation suggests that keeping the temperature of your bedroom below 70 degrees could help you to achieve a more restful and recuperative sleep. Keeping your room warm could cause you to toss and turn in the night, needing to readjust your covers, roll over, or even get up in the middle of the night to make temperature changes. Cooling things down could get you warmed up for a great sleep each night.

Lastly, it has been found that if you're using your bed for waking activities like work, watching television, eating, or other activities that keep the brain stimulated, it could disrupt your sleep. If your body doesn't see your bed solely as a place for rest and relaxation, it could keep that melatonin from forming. Try to keep all waking activities to other places of the house so that when you lie down in bed, your brain is primed and ready for sleep.

If you're finding that you're having trouble keeping yourself from snacking, take a look at your sleep schedule. If you have some trouble getting and/or staying asleep, try some of the above to see if that helps you to get that rest that your body unquestionably needs.

Too Many Visuals of Food

Visuals of food are everywhere. Advertisements, pictures and videos on social media, television, magazines, newspapers, etc. Anywhere you can read or watch, there are visuals and descriptions of food that can make it difficult to resist having some food. Those visuals are meant to make you hungry, so you'll buy those products. The thing is, when you're trying to keep to a more restrictive regimen, that can cause you some problems.

One way to curb this natural response to stimuli, is to change your actions when it kicks in. When you find yourself getting hungry because of an advertisement, picture, or other media, make it a point to do something else. Think of something you would rather do when that forced hunger sneaks up on you like reading, drawing, or even just chewing a piece of sugar-free gum. These could be helpful responses when things like tantalizing videos of food make you want to eat everything in the refrigerator or order out.

The goal is to avoid a situation in which you feel like you need to snack repeatedly throughout the day. However, if you do need to snack throughout the day, your absolute best bet is vegetables and fruits. Snacking on things that have a low carb and calorie count is perfect when you just need a little boost in your day, and it won't throw off your progress with a keto regimen. It can be hard, though, to push yourself into grabbing for something like fruits or vegetables if you're used to grabbing for something like candy or chips.

The best thing to do to ensure you're not in any danger of turning to candy or chips, is to keep them out of the house. In addition to this, prepare your snacks ahead of time so you can just grab and go. When you're feeling the urge to snack, having to prepare something while you're hungry can be a hassle and a deterrent. If the fruits and vegetables are all ready for you and prepared the way you need them to be, you can grab them, satiate the craving, and be on your way in no time!

It's so helpful to have these prepared when you need them, which is what makes it a golden rule for weight loss on keto!

Choose your Meal Before Going Out

Going on a diet can feel like punishment from time to time. With keto, it really is the changing of your lifestyle. This means that it is best done when you see it as your new everyday regimen. If you do it with the concept that this is how you eat, regardless of any time limits, it will be easier to acclimate and adjust to the changes you'll be making. However, part of life is going out to eat with friends and family.

You may have found that it seems impossible to lose weight when you go out to eat on a semi-regular basis, even though you might be trying hard to make the right choices on the menu. Let's examine this, shall we? When we go out to eat, it's customary to get an appetizer, a drink that isn't water, an entrée with two sides, and dessert is always offered. The problem with this is that the entrée and sides are generally 2-3 times a typical serving size for that type of food. You are generally taking on 2-3 times more food than would be recommended in a sitting, if you were to clear your plates at dinner.

On top of this overabundance, it is typical for the most delicious and creative menu options to involve more carbohydrates and bad fats than you typically want to take in in a sitting. It can seem like, when you go out to eat, the deck is stacked against you. In spite of this, there are some steps you can take to ensure you don't overeat and that you don't make the wrong choices when you go.

Before you go out to dinner, use the computer or your smartphone and visit the website of the establishment you'll be attending. Generally, there will be a section of the website that provides a PDF or image of their menu. Looking over the menu before you head out the restaurant can give you an idea of the appetizers that they offer, so you can have a strong voice in directing your party toward that option. Spinach artichoke dip is usually an appetizer staple in American restaurants and the kitchen may be able to make substitutions for the tortilla strips that typically come with it, like celery or another option on their menu.

You can also select your entrée and side options prior to going to the restaurant. Doing so will eliminate the need to look through the menu and the possibility of your making a rash decision.

Going into the restaurant with the express intent of grabbing the salmon with a side of steamed asparagus and a garden salad, is your best bet to actually end up with those items at your table. If you're flipping through the menu and see the crispy chicken sandwich, your likelihood of getting a low-carb option to appeal to you after that is significantly lower.

Taking control of what you order before you go will help you to maintain all the progress you've worked hard to make in your regimen. There is another way to help you exercise more self-control when you go to the restaurant as well. When you order your food, you can ask that half of the portion be boxed up before it gets brought to the table. This will ensure that you're not eating the entirety of what is brought out to you and will be more cost-effective. It is true that you can order half-portions of many entrees at restaurants, but you will often find that the price for those is more than half of the entrée cost.

The above are essential tips for being able to enjoy a nice meal out with friends and family. Being able to go out to eat while staying on track and saving money are all huge benefits that will help you to achieve longevity on a regimen such as this! Give it a shot and see how this method serves you.

<u>Stick to the List</u>

When you head to the grocery store after starting a new regimen or diet like keto, you will find that habit will take the wheel from time to time. Occasionally, you will find yourself in the chip or snack aisle when you hadn't intended to end up there. Not having a grocery list when you end up in these places unexpectedly can lead to purchases of items we don't need, and neglect of the items that we do need.

Properly structuring your grocery shopping list is a large part of planning your grocery trip. When your grocery list is properly structured, you end up covering a lot of your bases in one fell swoop. That proper structure can be the key to ensuring that:

- You get in and out of the grocery store in a timely manner
- You save money by getting exactly what you need, nothing more and nothing less
- You limit the number of items coming into your home that aren't conducive to your success
- You do not waste any food by having items that will preclude you from using the ones you should be using

Properly structuring your grocery list depends largely on the layout of your grocery store. It is a favorite tactic of mine to list the categories on my shopping list in the same order in which I pass through those sections in the grocery store. This way, my grocery list also serves as a map that gives me the most direct route through the store. Let's take a look at a sample list that could see you through your next trip, shall we?

<u>Produce</u>
Apples
Bell Peppers
Cauliflower
Celery
Cilantro
Cucumbers
Grape Tomatoes
Lemons

<u>Deli/Seafood</u>
Muenster Cheese
Hummus
Salmon
Sliced Turkey

<u>Canned/Dry Goods</u>
Bone Broth
Coconut Flour
Diced Tomatoes
Nuts

<u>Meat</u>
Chicken Breasts
Ground Beef
Ground Turkey

<u>Frozen</u>
Broccoli
Spinach
Stir Fry Vegetables

<u>Dairy Case</u>
Eggs
Plain Yogurt
Shredded Cheese

This is an example of a list that outlines what is in each section and would quickly get you through a grocery store. Getting to know your local grocery store and its layout could help you to establish a list and path to help you with success. When you know where everything is, you know what sections to avoid. You know what you need to go for, you set your sights on that, and it's hard for much of anything else to come into the equation without your say-so!

This is what it looks like to take complete control of your shopping experience and outcome. You don't need to be the victim of eerily relevant marketing schemes to get you to buy food items you do not need, and which will not contribute to the healthier, freer lifestyle you're working toward by starting a ketogenic regimen. Take a look at the list of items you need from the grocery store this week and do your best to recall what section comes first when you walk through the door at the store. Write that down and try to think of what section comes next. Continue this until you know what basic sections, you'll need to use to break down your grocery list. The good thing about this process is that you'll only need to do it once for every trip you take to that particular grocery store.

This method is a great way to help you stick to your grocery list. This will ensure that you're getting in and out in a reasonable amount of time and you can be sure that you're not coming away with any items that will only make it harder to stick to your diet as you get through your week!

Bonus Tip: make sure you never go to the store on an empty stomach! If you're anything like me, you get really creative about the foods you'd like to eat when you're hungry. Being creative at the grocery store can get very expensive and very fattening much more quickly than you might imagine. Save yourself money and carb intake by having a healthy snack before embarking on your grocery shopping trip!

Chapter 5: Control Weight Loss and

Get Energy

Autophagy is a bodily process whereby cells are broken down and recycled through your system. You've heard that the body sheds cells in your body and makes room for fresh, new cells. This is a heavily simplified explanation for what autophagy is, but it gives you an idea of what it is. As you get older, however, this process isn't as fast as it once was, and this leaves us with the bodily effects of aging.

Let's take a look at what some of the effects of having slowed autophagy are. Because autophagy is the body's way of keeping healthy, effective cells in your body, there are endless things that can be affected if your autophagy process has slowed in your body. Some of the things you could experience are sluggishness, dull skin, sagging skin, increased infections or illness, general aging, and more. What we are attempting to do when we work to speed up autophagy is essentially halting or slowing the aging process in the body.

If the body is aging more slowly and the cells are healthy, your immune response, your skin, your internal systems, and your vitality will all be at an optimum or peak condition. Stopping the aging process has been the goal of man for centuries, so have we finally found it? Many scientific and medical sources tell us that this is as close as we've ever come, and that protecting and speeding up our autophagy is the answer to staying young, vital, and healthy for many years!

So, what is the best way to monitor and improve this process? There are a number of factors that can go a long way toward helping you achieve this accelerated autophagy that you need in order to halt aging and boost your energy levels! The two most crucial elements will help you to keep your body in ketosis and will help you to control your weight loss and energy levels with little to no difficulty! Let's take a look at those two key components now and break them down so you can put them to work for you in your life.

Intermittent Fasting

Intermittent fasting, as its name implies, is a regimen of fasting for specific periods of time, on a schedule that works best for you. This is a fluid process, so you can change it as you need to do so, and you can make adjustments as you learn more about the process, how it makes you feel, and what works best with your daily regimen. When you take on intermittent fasting, it is important to note that it does not put any restrictions on the *types* of foods you can eat. This means that you can do intermittent fasting, while still ensuring that everything you eat is in line with a keto diet.

Intermittent fasting means that you will go from periods in which you will eat nothing, to periods during with there are no limits on what you should be eating. As previously mentioned, there are myriad ways in which you can structure this, so don't feel like you need to stick to any specific structure, unless that works best for you. When you're picking your method and your schedule for intermittent fasting, it's also important to have your goals in mind for it.

In order to appropriately choose goals for this, you'll need to know what things intermittent fasting can do for you. You can't set goals appropriately if you're not doing things that will realistically accomplish those things, right? So, let's take a look at the things that you can expect to come from something like an intermittent fasting regimen.

Weight Loss – There are a number of studies that show us that eating on this schedule can adjust your metabolism and help you to burn excess body fat. Generally speaking, when doing an intermittent fasting schedule will mean that you eat fewer meals overall. Unless you're working hard to make up those lost calories, your body will be thriving on a lower intake, which will deplete the fat reserves in your body.

Eating less throughout the day lowers the insulin levels in your body, raises growth hormone levels, and increases levels of norepinephrine. All of these things contribute to and increase the breakdown of excess fat within the body. It is because of this that your metabolism increases. Those who do intermittent fasting can expect and increase in metabolic rate of up to 14%, which is quite the metabolic overhaul.

This is a really great mechanism of intermittent fasting because it not only lowers the number of calories you're taking in throughout the day, it increases your capacity to process the calories that you're taking on. Additionally, your body is working harder, so it's actually burning more calories throughout the day. This gives you an ideal ratio of calories in, to calories out, contributing to some pretty phenomenal weight loss results!

Reduced Risk of Built-Up Insulin Resistance (Type 2 Diabetes) – Type 2 Diabetes, or increased insulin resistance, is an increasingly more prevalent affliction in today's world. As the diet of the everyday person continues to evolve to include more carbohydrates, as the body continues to depend on sugar for energy, and as activity levels drop, the risk is as high as it's ever been. There are ways, however, of avoiding this illness and of keeping your body healthy.

We mentioned earlier that your body will be producing lower levels of insulin as you eat less throughout the day. Since insulin production is a natural response to food intake, that response is lessened when fewer meals are eaten over time. Because your body is producing less insulin and producing less of it, your resistance to insulin will be far less aggressive.

Like with any chemical in the body, increased amounts will lower the body's capacity to be affected by it. Furthermore, reducing one's exposure to those chemicals will reduce the body's resistance to them as well. Backing down the insulin production inside your body with an intermittent fasting regimen, according to studies conducted on the matter and reported on by medical journals, can greatly reduce your risk of Type 2 Diabetes.

Studies indicate that the blood sugar of the average person who is on an intermittent fasting regimen was reduced by 3%-6%. Insulin levels in that same person were found to be reduced by as much as 20%-31%. In addition to this, rats who were put on an intermittent fasting regimen were found to have protection against kidney damage, which is one of the most severe complications connected to diabetes.

Improved Heart Health —In the end of the 20th century, heart disease moved to the top of the charts for leading causes of death in the Western world. There are many things linked to heart disease, but diet and exercise are two of the most talked-about. It is true that improving the things you eat can help your body to keep your cardiovascular system primed, working, and strong. It seems, however, that intermittent fasting, could give us the leg up we need to put the risk of cardiovascular disease firmly out of our minds. There are a good number of aspects or "risk factors" that are taken into consideration when it comes to heart disease. These include blood pressure, cholesterol, blood triglycerides, blood sugar levels, and more. These are based on many animal studies, but it does give us an idea of things we can monitor personally until more, human-based conclusions can be made by medical outfits.

The good thing about these aspects of our health, is that they can all be linked to the foods we eat, and our metabolism of those foods. By changing the quality of the foods we're taking in, lowering the amount of food that our bodies have to handle, our bodies have fewer of these problems to handle. Thanks to these mitigations and changes, the burden on your cardiovascular system is lessened significantly, thus improving your chances of avoiding heart disease.

Improved Brain Health – Various aspects of the metabolic processes are known to be essential to the health and function of the brain. Several studies conducted showed that participants experienced an increased growth of new nerve cells while on a regimen of intermittent fasting. That production should greatly benefit the overall health and functionality of the brain.

Studies conducted also show us that participants experienced increased production of a hormone called BDNF or Brain-Derived Neurotrophic Factor. The deficiency of this hormone has been linked with neurological and psychological disorders. Depression is one such issue that has been linked to a deficiency in BDNF.

Another study tells us that the fortitude and durability of the brain increased due to an intermittent fasting regimen. This fortitude protected against brain damage caused as a result of a stroke that occurred in the participant. This could mean that the brain's resilience can be increased over time as a result of what and when we eat. Overall brain health and well-being seem to be linked to diet and regimen.

Higher Energy Level – At this point, there is no question as to whether or not a ketogenic diet will give you more energy. This is because your body is currently working off of the stores of fat in your body, as well as the fat you're diligently giving it at every appropriate mealtime. Piggybacking intermittent fasting onto this process and giving your body more time to work off of those reserves gives your body more, longer-lasting energy that you will feel within a short time of adopting the regimen.

Your body is expending less of the energy it's getting from that constant burn. Normally, your body would be using a portion of the energy in your body to metabolize and break down the foods you give it. When you stop needing to give your body as much food in a given period, that leaves excess energy for you to use throughout your day.

What you will do with all the extra energy you have as a result of these practices is up to you! Exercise will be easier than ever before and won't leave you feeling sluggish from having expended so much of your energy. You will have more time in your day to dedicate to the things you want, and the lifestyle you want to live.

Fewer Interruptions for Food in Your Day – Shopping, cooking, meal preparation, and eating are all activities that take up a large amount of time. When you have to worry about less of each of these things, there's more time in your day for other things that matter to you and which you would like to be doing.

This item feeds back into our previous item, having more time to do more of the things that you want to do, and which excite you. Having more hours in the day is one of those pipe dreams that people mention. This is the genie in the lamp, giving you that extra time in the day that so many of us need. Let's make the best of that extra time we have and live a life we love living.

A Reduced Risk of Cancer – Cancer is becoming more of a prevalent problem in modern society and poses a threat to our health and livelihood. Being able to cure or avoid it is something modern scientists are currently striving for.

While there is no definitive answer as to one root cause or cure as of yet, we do know that cancer cells thrive in an environment with high glucose levels. On a diet that is focused around primarily burning sugar, the glucose levels in your body increase every time you eat something. Switching to something like a keto regimen, then cutting down the number of times you're eating throughout the week, gives your body less glucose. Those cells have less of that nutrient on which to thrive.

While this isn't completely concrete proof, the inclination of cancer cells to thrive in a high-sugar environment is certainly a motivating reason to reduce or cut that element from your internal environment. Your microbiome will thank you and lessening risk factors for such a serious illness is unquestionably an item in the positive category.

Easier to Stick to Than Dieting – Because the types of foods you can eat are not dictated by this regimen, it can be an easier transition. Doing an intermittent fast with the food approved for a ketogenic regimen, your body will acclimate to the space between meals with ease. Your body will have enough energy to get from meal to meal, and you will find that the act of fasting itself will give you more energy as well.

Many diets and regimens are often a setup for failure, but a ketogenic regimen and intermittent fasting are two that can be done on an indefinite basis, and with undeniable results. In addition to this, there are several different methods by which to go about intermittent fasting, so it really is all about whatever works best for you and your body. Pick a regimen that fits in with the times and things that fit in with the lifestyle you're working to achieve, and everything will fall into place as you achieve normalcy on those regimens.
Essential Chemical Processes Changed Within Your Body – As we've discussed in this chapter, a great many of the processes, hormones, and cells in your body will be affected by a regimen like this. Hormone production will be more ideal, your cells will be renewed and cleaned out at an accelerated rate (this is the autophagy we talked about speeding up), and your body will be more able to keep up with the daily effort of keeping you moving.

With lower insulin production, increased hormone production in the brain, lower usage of glucose, and so much more, the body is running as efficiently on as little food as is possible. This is the ideal situation for your health, your wallet, your time, and your life. Every chemical process in your body that is affected by the intake of food, can be positively affected with the addition of a ketogenic intermittent fast regimen.

Minimized Inflammation and Oxidative Stress – Inflammation and Oxidative Stress have a lot of causes, but those who have switched to intermittent fasting saw a reduction in both. Studies tell us that inflammation in various parts of the body can lead to more serious, albeit common illnesses in the body.

By eating foods that have less of a tendency to inflame the systems within your body and limiting food intake to the times specified for your intermittent fasting, you are giving your body the time to settle any inflammation between meals.

Oxidative stress and inflammation both play a role in things like illness, chronic illness, and aging. By limiting these two processes, you can significantly improve your chances of living a longer, healthier life. Studies indicate that you can stay healthier and give yourself more time to enjoy the things that you want out of life by reducing these two processes in the body.

Reduced Risk of Neurodegenerative Diseases – Alzheimer's currently has no known cure. However, in studies conducted on rats on an intermittent fasting regimen, researchers found that intermittent fasting had a connection to delaying the onset and minimizing the severity of symptoms in Alzheimer's patients.

Further animal studies show us that a regimen on intermittent fasting could also protect against Parkinson's or Huntington's disease. More research in humans is needed to tell us if this is something, we can do to combat the diseases, but undertaking such a regimen could be the head start someone needs if they're genetically predisposed to such a condition.

Now that we've discussed the potential benefits of doing an intermittent fast while on your ketogenic regimen, let's talk about the various ways in which you could structure your fasting schedule. This is based entirely on what you want and will not affect the positive results that you can get from it, regardless of which decision you make.

The first way to go about intermittent fasting is on a daily regimen. This is characterized by a 16-hour fast, which is followed by an 8-hour period in which you take in your meals. The benefit of doing this every day is that it's a lot easier to acclimate. You won't have to think about which day you're on, what time you should eat based on the date, and the like. You'll only have to keep an eye on the clock and eat at the times you set at the outset.

This layout for your regimen is a suggestion, and the timing itself is up to you, but here is a sample of your week, laid out with this regimen. If you're working third shift or you have a reason why you would need to begin eating earlier in the day, you can adjust the timing so it still works out to 16 hours of fasting, to eight hours of regular eating, on an alternating basis. If you're having difficulty with achieving a balance on this regimen, speak with your physician about how you could work your way into a regimen that fits your schedule, your nutritional needs, and your expectations.

Daily Fasting Plan

Monday

12:00 AM – 12:00 PM –
Fasting
12:00- PM – 8:00 PM –
Eating regularly
8:00 PM – 12:00 AM
Fasting

Tuesday

12:00 AM – 12:00 PM –
Fasting
12:00- PM – 8:00 PM –
Eating regularly
8:00 PM – 12:00 AM
Fasting

Wednesday

12:00 AM – 12:00 PM –
Fasting
12:00- PM – 8:00 PM –
Eating regularly
8:00 PM – 12:00 AM
Fasting

Thursday

12:00 AM – 12:00 PM –
Fasting
12:00- PM – 8:00 PM –
Eating regularly
8:00 PM – 12:00 AM
Fasting

Friday

12:00 AM – 12:00 PM –
Fasting
12:00- PM – 8:00 PM –
Eating regularly
8:00 PM – 12:00 AM
Fasting

Saturday

12:00 AM – 12:00 PM –
Fasting
12:00- PM – 8:00 PM –
Eating regularly
8:00 PM – 12:00 AM
Fasting

Typically, when you adopt this regimen for your intermittent fasting, you will have a lunch at around noon, a healthy snack, and dinner at around six at night. Now, if you wish to eat more than this or if you feel like you might need to take on more fat and protein to get you through your next fast, then you are encouraged to do so. It is advised that you keep your macronutrient guidelines in mind when you make your food choices between fasts, and it's advised that you don't go overboard with the size of your meals and snacks. If you feel the need to go overboard with your meals and snacks between fasts, it could mean that you need to add protein and fat in the right ratios, so your body has enough to work with.

Pay attention to the foods that will give you a good fat to protein ratio, your minerals, vitamins, and your water intake.

As long as all those things are kept where they should be, your regimen should go as smoothly as you need it to. If you find that you're having difficulty with keeping on this pattern and you feel like you're keeping all of the above in mind, you may want to speak with your physician about what changes or supplements you can make to your regimen so it suits all of your needs.

The next type of fasting plan is to take one fast each week, which lasts for a period of 24 hours. This means that you will eat for the first four hours in one day of the week, then fast straight through until noon the next day. This might be a little bit harder for some to do, as going an entire day without eating is a not a typical behavior for the everyday person. If you want to work up to this, it is certainly something to work toward. You can go through your entire day, not having to worry about preparing a single meal! Let's take a look at what your week could look like if you adopted this regimen.

<u>Once Weekly Fast</u>

<u>Monday</u>
12:00 AM – 8:00 AM –
Fasting (sleeping)
8:00 AM – 12:00 PM –
Eating Regularly
12:00 PM – 12:00 AM -
Fasting

<u>Tuesday</u>
12:00 AM – 12:00 PM –
Fasting (sleeping)
12:00 PM – 12:00 AM –
Eating Regularly

<u>Wednesday</u>
12:00 AM – 8:00 AM –
Fasting (sleeping)
8:00 AM – 12:00 AM –
Eating Regularly

<u>Thursday</u>
12:00 AM – 8:00 AM –
Fasting (sleeping)
8:00 AM – 12:00 AM –
Eating Regularly

<u>Friday</u>
12:00 AM – 8:00 AM –
Fasting (sleeping)
8:00 AM – 12:00 AM –
Eating Regularly

<u>Saturday</u>
12:00 AM – 8:00 AM –
Fasting (sleeping)
8:00 AM – 12:00 AM –
Eating Regularly

It is typically recommended that you don't eat anything within 2-3 hours of going to sleep, as your body won't be making use of the food you're putting into it. Your body will still be burning fat as you sleep, so this is less of a concern than it might be otherwise. However, eating directly before bed or at late hours of the evening could lead to an energy spike, which could make it more difficult for you to sleep.

That being said, this regimen is particularly helpful if you're planning on taking a day trip somewhere. You can structure your week so that fast occurs on that trip, which would save you time when making stops, as well as a considerable amount of money. Eating out while traveling can be a huge drain on the budget, so it helps to avoid that!

Whatever day you decide to pick for your intermittent fast, it is recommended that you allow yourself those four hours in the beginning of the day on which you start. It will make it easier for you to get through that first day, as opposed to having nothing to eat at all as you undertake those next 24 hours of fasting.

You may want to take this method into consideration if you decide to go for the next method of intermittent fasting, which is a little bit more intensive. We're going to take a look at a regimen that allows you to alternate full days of fasting, so your body is running on as little fuel as possible within a one-week period.

These are laid out in a progression, as these methods get a little bit steeper in terms of commitment to the regimen. In a moment, we will talk more about how to structure a progression that will get you closer to achieving this sort of regimen, as going so right out of the gate might be a little bit of a shock to those who are used to eating on a very regular basis.

As we have pointed out about the other fasting schedules, the more time you spend fasting is the less time through which you will need to buy, prepare, and eat food. More of your time and energy is expended on the things in your life that are the most important.

Alternating Full-Day Fasting Schedule

Monday
12:00 AM – 8:00 AM –
Fasting (sleeping)
8:00 AM – 12:00 PM –
Eating Regularly
12:00 PM – 12:00 AM -
Fasting

Tuesday
12:00 AM – 12:00 PM –
Fasting (sleeping)
12:00 PM – 12:00 AM –
Eating Regularly

Wednesday
12:00 AM – 8:00 AM –
Fasting (sleeping)
8:00 AM – 12:00 PM –
Eating Regularly
12:00 PM – 12:00 AM -
Fasting

Thursday
12:00 AM – 12:00 PM –
Fasting (sleeping)
12:00 PM – 12:00 AM –
Eating Regularly

Friday
12:00 AM – 8:00 AM –
Fasting (sleeping)
8:00 AM – 12:00 PM –
Eating Regularly
12:00 PM – 12:00 AM -
Fasting

Saturday
12:00 AM – 12:00 PM –
Fasting (sleeping)
12:00 PM – 12:00 AM –
Eating Regularly

Employing a schedule like this gives you a lot of time during which you won't need to be concerned with things like eating or preparing meals. This leaves you having to prepare only 12 meals for your week, plus snack. When you compare this to the 21 meals that we generally need to plan over the course of a week, this really is a huge time and money saver when it's done correctly.

As we mentioned, however, it can be hard to jump into a regimen as intensive as this one with no lead-up. Let's take a look at how we can make a plan that could, within a few weeks, get us ready to adopt a regimen of this sort without being a shock or a burden on the system!

As noted for the previous layouts, this is a suggestion and it can be altered for whatever best fits your dietary needs. Do not be afraid to take the reins and create a system or a schedule that is more to your liking. The most important part of figuring out a dietary regimen is you. You are the center of all of it and

the only reason to do any of this is to make a better life for you.
Don't be afraid to make changes so it's more of your own
program.

The brief rundown of the layout that is below will follow this
basic format:

Week 1: Daily Fasting

Week 2: Daily Fasting

Week 3: Weekly Fasting

Week 4: Weekly Fasting (Modified)

Week 5: Alternate Full-Day Fasting

Week 6: Alternate Full-Day Fasting

Let's take a look at this on an expanded basis to give us a
clearer description of the schedules this would entail.

<u>Week 1: Daily Fasting</u>

<u>Monday</u>
12:00 AM – 12:00 PM –
Fasting
12:00- PM – 8:00 PM –
Eating regularly
8:00 PM – 12:00 AM
Fasting

<u>Tuesday</u>
12:00 AM – 12:00 PM –
Fasting
12:00- PM – 8:00 PM –
Eating regularly
8:00 PM – 12:00 AM
Fasting

<u>Wednesday</u>
12:00 AM – 12:00 PM –
Fasting
12:00- PM – 8:00 PM –
Eating regularly
8:00 PM – 12:00 AM
Fasting

<u>Thursday</u>
12:00 AM – 12:00 PM –
Fasting
12:00- PM – 8:00 PM –
Eating regularly
8:00 PM – 12:00 AM
Fasting

<u>Friday</u>
12:00 AM – 12:00 PM –
Fasting
12:00- PM – 8:00 PM –
Eating regularly
8:00 PM – 12:00 AM
Fasting

<u>Saturday</u>
12:00 AM – 12:00 PM –
Fasting
12:00- PM – 8:00 PM –
Eating regularly
8:00 PM – 12:00 AM
Fasting

<u>Sunday</u>

12:00 AM – 12:00 PM –
Fasting

12:00- PM – 8:00 PM –
Eating regularly

8:00 PM – 12:00 AM
Fasting

<u>Week 2: Daily Fasting</u>

<u>Monday</u>

12:00 AM – 12:00 PM –
Fasting

12:00- PM – 8:00 PM –
Eating regularly

8:00 PM – 12:00 AM
Fasting

<u>Tuesday</u>

12:00 AM – 12:00 PM –
Fasting

12:00- PM – 8:00 PM –
Eating regularly

8:00 PM – 12:00 AM
Fasting

<u>Wednesday</u>

12:00 AM – 12:00 PM –
Fasting

12:00- PM – 8:00 PM –
Eating regularly

8:00 PM – 12:00 AM
Fasting

<u>Thursday</u>

12:00 AM – 12:00 PM –
Fasting

12:00- PM – 8:00 PM –
Eating regularly

8:00 PM – 12:00 AM
Fasting

<u>Friday</u>
12:00 AM – 12:00 PM –
Fasting
12:00- PM – 8:00 PM –
Eating regularly
8:00 PM – 12:00 AM
Fasting

<u>Saturday</u>
12:00 AM – 12:00 PM –
Fasting
12:00- PM – 8:00 PM –
Eating regularly
8:00 PM – 12:00 AM
Fasting

<u>Sunday</u>
12:00 AM – 12:00 PM –
Fasting
12:00- PM – 8:00 PM –
Eating regularly
8:00 PM – 12:00 AM
Fasting

<u>Week 3: Weekly Fast</u>

<u>Monday</u>
12:00 AM – 8:00 AM –
Fasting (sleeping)
8:00 AM – 12:00 PM –
Eating Regularly
12:00 PM – 12:00 AM -
Fasting

<u>Tuesday</u>
12:00 AM – 12:00 PM –
Fasting
12:00 PM – 12:00 AM –
Eating Regularly

<u>Wednesday</u>
12:00 AM – 8:00 AM –
Fasting (sleeping)
8:00 AM – 12:00 AM –
Eating Regularly

<u>Thursday</u>
12:00 AM – 8:00 AM –
Fasting (sleeping)
8:00 AM – 12:00 AM –
Eating Regularly

<u>Friday</u>
12:00 AM – 8:00 AM –
Fasting (sleeping)
8:00 AM – 12:00 AM –
Eating Regularly

<u>Saturday</u>
12:00 AM – 8:00 AM –
Fasting (sleeping)
8:00 AM – 12:00 AM –
Eating Regularly

<u>Sunday</u>
12:00 AM – 8:00 AM –
Fasting (sleeping)
8:00 AM – 12:00 AM –
Eating Regularly

Week 4: Weekly Fast (Modified)

Monday
12:00 AM – 8:00 AM –
Fasting (sleeping)
8:00 AM – 12:00 PM –
Eating Regularly
12:00 PM – 12:00 AM -
Fasting

Tuesday
12:00 AM – 12:00 PM –
Fasting
12:00 PM – 12:00 AM –
Eating Regularly

Wednesday
12:00 AM – 8:00 AM –
Fasting (sleeping)
8:00 AM – 12:00 AM –
Eating Regularly

Thursday
12:00 AM – 8:00 AM –
Fasting (sleeping)
8:00 AM – 12:00 AM –
Eating Regularly

Friday
12:00 AM – 8:00 AM –
Fasting (sleeping)
8:00 AM – 12:00 PM –
Eating Regularly
12:00 PM – 12:00 AM -
Fasting

Saturday
12:00 AM – 12:00 PM –
Fasting
12:00 PM – 12:00 AM –
Eating Regularly

<u>Sunday</u>
12:00 AM – 8:00 AM –
Fasting (sleeping)
8:00 AM – 12:00 AM –
Eating Regularly

<u>Week 5: Alternate Full-Day Fasting</u>

<u>Monday</u>
12:00 AM – 8:00 AM –
Fasting (sleeping)
8:00 AM – 12:00 PM –
Eating Regularly
12:00 PM – 12:00 AM -
Fasting

<u>Tuesday</u>
12:00 AM – 12:00 PM –
Fasting
12:00 PM – 12:00 AM –
Eating Regularly

<u>Wednesday</u>
12:00 AM – 8:00 AM –
Fasting (sleeping)
8:00 AM – 12:00 PM –
Eating Regularly
12:00 PM – 12:00 AM -
Fasting

<u>Thursday</u>
12:00 AM – 12:00 PM –
Fasting
12:00 PM – 12:00 AM –
Eating Regularly

<u>Friday</u>
12:00 AM – 8:00 AM –
Fasting (sleeping)
8:00 AM – 12:00 PM –
Eating Regularly
12:00 PM – 12:00 AM -
Fasting

<u>Saturday</u>
12:00 AM – 12:00 PM –
Fasting
12:00 PM – 12:00 AM –
Eating Regularly

<u>Sunday</u>
12:00 AM – 8:00 AM –
Fasting (sleeping)
8:00 AM – 12:00 PM –
Eating Regularly
12:00 PM – 12:00 AM -
Fasting

Week 6: Alternate Full-Day Fasting

<u>Monday</u>
12:00 AM – 8:00 AM –
Fasting (sleeping)
8:00 AM – 12:00 PM –
Eating Regularly
12:00 PM – 12:00 AM -
Fasting

<u>Tuesday</u>
12:00 AM – 12:00 PM –
Fasting
12:00 PM – 12:00 AM –
Eating Regularly

<u>Wednesday</u>
12:00 AM – 8:00 AM –
Fasting (sleeping)
8:00 AM – 12:00 PM –
Eating Regularly
12:00 PM – 12:00 AM -
Fasting

<u>Thursday</u>
12:00 AM – 12:00 PM –
Fasting
12:00 PM – 12:00 AM –
Eating Regularly

<u>Friday</u>
12:00 AM – 8:00 AM –
Fasting
8:00 AM – 12:00 PM –
Eating Regularly
12:00 PM – 12:00 AM -
Fasting

<u>Saturday</u>
12:00 AM – 12:00 PM –
Fasting
12:00 PM – 12:00 AM –
Eating Regularly

<u>Sunday</u>

12:00 AM – 8:00 AM –
Fasting (sleeping)

8:00 AM – 12:00 PM –
Eating Regularly

12:00 PM – 12:00 AM -
Fasting

With schedules that are similar to the above 6-week plan, you should be able to create or adopt a plan that can help you to get to the most energy-efficient mode of operations possible for you, your body, and the lifestyle you wish to live. Take a look at how you might be able to adapt the schedule above so that in six weeks, you could be running as lean as this. Make sure you document the changes you make as you go from week to week as well.

Make note of what you ate and when, and how you felt throughout the day. If you notice that a new regimen change isn't serving you well enough, you can take a look back at the things that you've tried in the past. You can see what things worked for you, what didn't, if anything might have gone wrong, and how to move forward with the greatest possible rate of success!

Protein Cycling

Protein cycling is a method that can be added to your fasting regimen to give you a little extra fat-burning boost. The principle behind it is that autophagy is sparked and accelerated by intermittent fasting, and alternating days of higher and lowered protein intake. The lowered protein intake in your body causes your cells to go into a shortage control mode that causes them to renew and clean out with a rapid pace.

It is not recommended to do this particular thing for a sustained period time, but a couple of weeks here and there will give you a good dose of autophagy acceleration that will keep you looking youthful and healthy! Because it is not recommended to go very high on your protein intake with a ketogenic regimen, it's a good idea to decide what your "high" and "low" amounts of protein will be, how to figure that into your meal planning, and how that will fit in with your intermittent fasting regimen.

Let's lay out the 6-week intermittent fast with those "high" and "low" protein days to give you an idea of how best to incorporate it into your regimen! This will be laid out on the next page so you can see what that would look like.

<u>Week 1: Daily Fasting</u>

<u>Monday "High" Protein</u>
12:00 AM – 12:00 PM –
Fasting
12:00- PM – 8:00 PM –
Eating regularly
8:00 PM – 12:00 AM
Fasting

<u>Tuesday "Low" Protein</u>
12:00 AM – 12:00 PM –
Fasting
12:00- PM – 8:00 PM –
Eating regularly
8:00 PM – 12:00 AM
Fasting

<u>Wednesday "High" Protein</u>
12:00 AM – 12:00 PM –
Fasting
12:00- PM – 8:00 PM –
Eating regularly
8:00 PM – 12:00 AM
Fasting

<u>Thursday "Low" Protein</u>
12:00 AM – 12:00 PM –
Fasting
12:00- PM – 8:00 PM –
Eating regularly
8:00 PM – 12:00 AM
Fasting

<u>Friday "High" Protein</u>
12:00 AM – 12:00 PM –
Fasting
12:00- PM – 8:00 PM –
Eating regularly
8:00 PM – 12:00 AM
Fasting

<u>Saturday "Low" Protein</u>
12:00 AM – 12:00 PM –
Fasting
12:00- PM – 8:00 PM –
Eating regularly
8:00 PM – 12:00 AM
Fasting

Sunday "High" Protein

12:00 AM – 12:00 PM – Fasting

12:00- PM – 8:00 PM – Eating regularly

8:00 PM – 12:00 AM Fasting

Week 2: Daily Fasting

Monday "High" Protein

12:00 AM – 12:00 PM – Fasting

12:00- PM – 8:00 PM – Eating regularly

8:00 PM – 12:00 AM Fasting

Tuesday "Low" Protein

12:00 AM – 12:00 PM – Fasting

12:00- PM – 8:00 PM – Eating regularly

8:00 PM – 12:00 AM Fasting

Wednesday "High" Protein

12:00 AM – 12:00 PM – Fasting

12:00- PM – 8:00 PM – Eating regularly

8:00 PM – 12:00 AM Fasting

Thursday "Low" Protein

12:00 AM – 12:00 PM – Fasting

12:00- PM – 8:00 PM – Eating regularly

8:00 PM – 12:00 AM Fasting

<u>Friday "High" Protein</u>
12:00 AM – 12:00 PM –
Fasting
12:00- PM – 8:00 PM –
Eating regularly
8:00 PM – 12:00 AM
Fasting

<u>Saturday "Low" Protein</u>
12:00 AM – 12:00 PM –
Fasting
12:00- PM – 8:00 PM –
Eating regularly
8:00 PM – 12:00 AM
Fasting

<u>Sunday "High" Protein</u>
12:00 AM – 12:00 PM –
Fasting
12:00- PM – 8:00 PM –
Eating regularly 8:00 PM –
12:00 AM Fasting

<u>Week 3: Weekly Fast (No Protein Cycling)</u>

<u>Monday</u>
12:00 AM – 8:00 AM –
Fasting (sleeping)
8:00 AM – 12:00 PM –
Eating Regularly
12:00 PM – 12:00 AM -
Fasting

<u>Tuesday</u>
12:00 AM – 12:00 PM –
Fasting
12:00 PM – 12:00 AM –
Eating Regularly

<u>Wednesday</u>
12:00 AM – 8:00 AM –
Fasting (sleeping)
8:00 AM – 12:00 AM –
Eating Regularly

<u>Thursday</u>
12:00 AM – 8:00 AM –
Fasting (sleeping)
8:00 AM – 12:00 AM –
Eating Regularly

<u>Friday</u>
12:00 AM – 8:00 AM –
Fasting (sleeping)
8:00 AM – 12:00 AM –
Eating Regularly

<u>Saturday</u>
12:00 AM – 8:00 AM –
Fasting (sleeping)
8:00 AM – 12:00 AM –
Eating Regularly

<u>Sunday</u>
12:00 AM – 8:00 AM –
Fasting (sleeping)
8:00 AM – 12:00 AM –
Eating Regularly

<u>Week 4: Weekly Fast (Modified) (No Protein Cycling)</u>

<u>Monday</u>
12:00 AM – 8:00 AM –
Fasting (sleeping)
8:00 AM – 12:00 PM –
Eating Regularly
12:00 PM – 12:00 AM -
Fasting

<u>Wednesday</u>
12:00 AM – 8:00 AM –
Fasting (sleeping)
8:00 AM – 12:00 AM –
Eating Regularly

<u>Tuesday</u>
12:00 AM – 12:00 PM –
Fasting
12:00 PM – 12:00 AM –
Eating Regularly

<u>Thursday</u>
12:00 AM – 8:00 AM –
Fasting (sleeping)
8:00 AM – 12:00 AM –
Eating Regularly

Friday

12:00 AM – 8:00 AM –
Fasting (sleeping)
8:00 AM – 12:00 PM –
Eating Regularly
12:00 PM – 12:00 AM -
Fasting

Saturday

12:00 AM – 12:00 PM –
Fasting
12:00 PM – 12:00 AM –
Eating Regularly

Sunday

12:00 AM – 8:00 AM –
Fasting (sleeping)
8:00 AM – 12:00 AM –
Eating Regularly

Week 5: Alternate Full-Day Fasting

Monday "Low" Protein

12:00 AM – 8:00 AM –
Fasting (sleeping)
8:00 AM – 12:00 PM –
Eating Regularly
12:00 PM – 12:00 AM -
Fasting

Tuesday "High" Protein

12:00 AM – 12:00 PM –
Fasting
12:00 PM – 12:00 AM –
Eating Regularly

Wednesday "Low" Protein

12:00 AM – 8:00 AM –
Fasting (sleeping)
8:00 AM – 12:00 PM –
Eating Regularly
12:00 PM – 12:00 AM -
Fasting

Thursday "High" Protein

12:00 AM – 12:00 PM –
Fasting
12:00 PM – 12:00 AM –
Eating Regularly

Friday "Low" Protein

12:00 AM – 8:00 AM –
Fasting (sleeping)
8:00 AM – 12:00 PM –
Eating Regularly
12:00 PM – 12:00 AM -
Fasting

Saturday "High" Protein

12:00 AM – 12:00 PM –
Fasting
12:00 PM – 12:00 AM –
Eating Regularly

Sunday "Low" Protein

12:00 AM – 8:00 AM –
Fasting (sleeping)
8:00 AM – 12:00 PM –
Eating Regularly 12:00 PM
– 12:00 AM - Fasting

Week 6: Alternate Full-Day Fasting

Monday "Low" Protein

12:00 AM – 8:00 AM –
Fasting (sleeping)
8:00 AM – 12:00 PM –
Eating Regularly
12:00 PM – 12:00 AM -
Fasting

Wednesday "Low" Protein

12:00 AM – 8:00 AM –
Fasting (sleeping)
8:00 AM – 12:00 PM –
Eating Regularly
12:00 PM – 12:00 AM -
Fasting

Tuesday "High" Protein

12:00 AM – 12:00 PM –
Fasting
12:00 PM – 12:00 AM –
Eating Regularly

Thursday "High" Protein

12:00 AM – 12:00 PM –
Fasting
12:00 PM – 12:00 AM –
Eating Regularly

<u>Friday "Low" Protein</u>
12:00 AM – 8:00 AM –
Fasting (sleeping)
8:00 AM – 12:00 PM –
Eating Regularly
12:00 PM – 12:00 AM -
Fasting

<u>Saturday "High" Protein</u>
12:00 AM – 12:00 PM –
Fasting
12:00 PM – 12:00 AM –
Eating Regularly

<u>Sunday "Low" Protein</u>
12:00 AM – 8:00 AM –
Fasting (sleeping)
8:00 AM – 12:00 PM –
Eating Regularly
12:00 PM – 12:00 AM -
Fasting

Following this example of a protein cycling plan could help you to wean onto an intermittent fast, while cycling protein for the fist and last two weeks. This will give your body that boosted autophagy, more vitality, ketosis, and all the good things the regimens laid out in this book can give you!

Be sure to document your methods and your progress so you can refer back to it. Making changes is great. However, knowing what you did that worked, what you did that didn't work, and everything in between, is the way to truly take control of your life. Writing down how you feel after each change you make can also help you to tell your doctor about all that you're doing and how it has affected you. This can give your doctor a much clearer perspective of how to help you to get the most out of your regimen.

Conclusion

Now that you have read *Keto Diet Lifestyle: Regain Confidence with the Ultimate Beginners Ketogenic Manual for Healthy Weight Loss Including 5+ Golden Rules and Recipes to Reboot Your Metabolism*, you have the tools and the information necessary to get you on the road to healthy, fast, sustainable weight loss. You know by now that the information you've gained by reading this book is about so much more than just weight loss. These are the tools to help you bring your body to its most optimum operating condition, its healthiest point, and its most energetic levels.

Utilizing the tools in this book in your everyday life, adopting the regimens laid out in these pages, and going forward putting all of this to use will be the ultimate step in the right direction for your health, well-being, energy, appearance, and lifestyle. Getting into ketosis and staying there will give you the energy you need to live the life of your dreams, and sustainability that will keep you going on this regimen for as long as you need or want to!

With crash diets, fad diets, and regimens not based in science, you get results that don't stay with you for any discernable amount of time. Success is possible on diets like that, but if the metabolism is harmed in the process, or if it's not re-trained, the progress will ultimately be very difficult to maintain for any duration.

You have the tools now to utilize a regimen that will make measurable steps in the right direction toward peak health for your body. The next step is to put together your grocery list, hit the grocery store, and get started living a healthy life where you are in complete control. Live a longer, healthier, more satisfied life by getting started today.

Recommend this book for those who wish to understand how a ketogenic diet works! It is great for those who wish to know what goes into working toward a healthier lifestyle, how to take control, and how to have the confidence to make it all work. Give your friends and family the real tools to use to build the life they want, too!

Intermittent Fasting Guide for Beginners:

By Patrick H. Smith

Disclaimer

The information listed by the author in this book is not intended, by the author or the publisher, to diagnose or treat any illnesses or diseases. The information herein is meant to provide helpful background and understanding of the topics and their theories. For diagnosis or treatment of any disease, illness, or medical problem, please contact a medical professional in that field. Neither the publisher nor the author is responsible or liable for any allergy or medical needs not addressed or exacerbated by the use of the information herein. No information in these pages should be construed as medical, legal, or psychological advice or instruction. All data is provided for informational purposes and does not constitute endorsement on behalf of the author or publisher.

Introduction

The following chapters will discuss the basics of developing an intermittent fasting program. This program is designed to help you lose unwanted weight, detox your organs and overall heal your body in hopes of transforming your life for the better. The majority of people wish to change their diets and relationships with food, this is to be expected in a society that loves fast foods and other processed goods. Even if you're not overweight many people still feel that their diets are unhealthy. If you feel like you are in need of a drastic change in dietary choices and physical health then you've found the right book.

So why would someone need an intermittent fasting practice? There are many reasons. While many have pressing health issues that must be addressed immediately, others may feel that their diets are simply unbalanced or in need of a reinvention. Some may just need a detox or cleanse to help reset their bodies and heal their organs. Some people may be fasting for religious or spiritual reasons. An intermittent fasting routine can help all three of these issues, showing that fasting is a versatile and effective means of attaining the life you wish to live.

In this book we aim to achieve our healthful goals. We strive to reach our desired weight, reconstruct our poor diets and feel great everyday through the transformative process of developing an intermittent fasting practice. This practice is a catalyst to overall health. Fasting has the ability to redesign our relationship with food, all the while allowing our organs to heal and for our bodies to shed excess weight. There are not only physical benefits, our minds with gain new perspectives on food and diet. With a new, positive outlook we can relieve stress and take control of our diets. These factors are crucial to transforming our lives for the better.

In a society that is technologically advanced and fast paced it is hard to make time to really think about our diets and relationship to foods. Fast food and junk foods are the quick option for a busy day, but this is a bad habit that is tough to break. Even though studies have shown that these sugary, processed foods are terrible for our health we are still subjected to advertising and marketing of these foods. The powerful corporations and companies have outwardly shown that they do not care about the health of the general public. These companies are well aware of their fault and seem to be making no effort to change their ways. This propagation of an unhealthy diet combined with a busy work schedule is the main culprit in our health problem today.

Convenience foods and the use of synthetic ingredients have caused the western world to lose sight of a natural diet. These detrimental ingredients have been linked to obesity, depression and diabetes. This is unacceptable. As the food industry became globalized these unhealthy eating habits are being promoted around the world. Less developed countries are being subjected to the same attacks on their dietary choices. This creates a wicked cycle as the major companies are not willing to give up their profits and the everyday citizen is forced to eat cheap, nutrient devoid foods. But what can be done to combat this atrocity?

While we are not trying to tackle the global food crisis in this book, we can offer ideas and practices to help the individual reclaim control over their diets. This is accomplished by choosing better foods, having a positive outlook and overall rebuilding our broken relationship with food. Intermittent fasting helps to promote all of these key factors. We must rebuild our idea of diet. Consider the food pyramid that many of us grew up with. This pyramid help unusually high standards for an average diet, offering a broad generalization that cannot be applied to everyone. This pyramid has since been abolished but still leaves its detrimental traces behind. No one concept is going to work for everyone, this is a key focus in this book. We cannot expect one diet plan or practice to fit to every lifestyle, intermittent fasting is great in that it is easily customizable to fit individual needs. The idea of three meals a day is an ill fated one, not everyone is going to need three huge meals. In the western world this is common practice. We are raised to believe that we must have three meals to survive, but his is just not true. Many are so accustomed to their three meals that if they miss one their bodies may react in adverse ways, causing stress and low energy. We must reconstruct these habits, and forged a path to a new diet, one that is working harmoniously with our bodies and specific individual needs. Intermittent fasting is the safest and most effective way to begin on this path.

With all the social issues facing our society it can be overwhelming to think that a lone individual can make a difference. But we assure you that you can change your body and environment. By taking back control of your diet you impact that world for the better. You will transform yourself into a healthy and positive person, which in turn may inspire others to do the same. You will alter your diet to be more local and healthy, thus taking away a small bit of power from the big companies and returning it to yourself. And overall you will prove to yourself that you do not have to be forced into a wicked cycle of terrible foods and habits, empowering yourself to do good in the world and do good for yourself.

A total self-transformation may seem to good to be true, but with intermittent fasting you can take control of your body and your life. With some dedication and discipline you can take the first few steps on a path to empowerment and initiate new habits and practices to improve your life. There are no excuses or reasons to not begin right away, the simple practice of intermittent fasting is simple to begin and requires little from you except an open mind and a willingness to change your life for the better. Let's begin this journey and dive into the world of intermittent fasting.

As you approach the beginning of your new transformative path be humbled that you have found a practice that is ancient and powerful. Fasting techniques have been used for centuries and centuries all throughout history and throughout many different cultures. These practice should be approached with humility and resect as you begin to transform your life. Having the respect for this practice will certainly carry over into your personal life as you develop respect for yourself and your body. This respect will go a long way in rebuilding our relationship with your body and with diet. Learning this respectful attitude is a transformative practice in itself. We must detox our bodies as well as our minds, shedding prejudice and narcissism. The practice of intermittent fasting is an individual one that aims to transform the individual as a whole. But this transformative power reaches beyond our bodies as we progress. We make a better impact on the environment, we improve the economy and even inspire those around us to find this respect.

We see here that the practice of intermittent fasting is a great personal endeavor but it also hold implications that reach the entire world around us. Let us begin on our transformative path. This is the first day of our new lives.

There are plenty of books on this subject on the market, thanks again for choosing this one! Every effort was made to ensure it is full of as much useful information as possible, please enjoy!

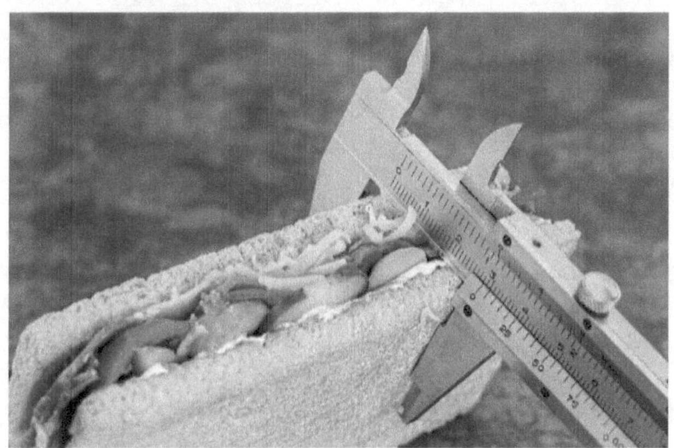

(Sandwich)

Chapter 1: What is Intermittent Fasting?

First things first, we need to find a suitable definition for intermittent fasting. While there are many ways to define a fast, a good basic definition is the intentional restriction of calories to promote healthful or religious progression. This restriction of caloric intake is the premise of fasting and its benefits. While many people think that to fast you must simply not eat, this is not quite true. Fasting does require you to go without food for a set duration of time, but there is much more to it than simply not eating, we need to develop our mindfulness and design a suitable diet when approaching an intermittent fasting practice. There needs to be careful contemplation and planning when we design our routine. The timeframes and limitations you personally set for your practice is just as important as the food itself. More on this in chapters to come.

Intermittent fasting has become quite popular in recent years as medical and fitness communities have adopted the practice into a healthy diet routine. This is good news for the health of the western world as science and medicine both validate a fasting routine as a healthful and effective practice. But fasting didn't just pop up out of nowhere to become the premier weight loss technique. Fasting, including intermittent fasting, has a rich cultural and spiritual history that spans all of written history and more than likely even before. This makes it obvious that there are many different variations on a fasting practice, as well as an abundant array of reasons to begin a fasting routine.

When you fast you may just be wanting to abstain from a certain food. Cutting out sweets for a month is technically a fast. You're fasting from sweets. This is common amongst religious holidays like Lent. Many people give up their cherished indulgence to prove their dedication to their religion and chose deity. This can be applied to a nonreligious context as well. Abstaining in any form can be viewed as a fast, although it's not a proper intermittent fasting diet. To form a full diet based around intermittent fasting we need to develop a routine and meal plan for us to adhere to. There are many different ways and reasons to fast, to reiterate, there is no one way that will work for everyone, so be open minded when developing your fasting regimen. As we begin to think about adopting fasting into our lives we need some context on the historical significance of fasting and how it has gone from ancient spiritual practice to popular fitness practice.

Historical Significance of Fasting

A quick glance at the lifestyles of our distant ancestors shows that fasting was a integral aspect of everyday life. In fact, not until just a couple hundred years ago fasting was readily practiced before becoming obscure and obsolete in the face of reasoning and science. These cultures used fasting for spiritual reasons as well as out of necessity. Whether it was an initiation into adulthood or a means to lengthen food rations, fasting has been an important part of humanity leading right up to today.

The current western culture places great emphases on appearances and convenience foods, our ancestors were not worried by such materialistic ideas. In these times health and spiritual communion were the hub of existence. Community and ritual were the focus, all while respecting nature and thriving within their means. This is far removed from our 'advanced' culture today. Consider the hunter-gatherer societies. These cultures would move from place to place hunting their food or foraging in the wild for it. Many experts agree that these people would often have hunts that were not successful, leading to calorie restricted days, or even weeks. This is essentially an intermittent fasting routine, although not as voluntary as the routines in the modern world.

Once agriculturally based societies were formed there was more consistency in food sources. This doesn't mean fasting wasn't implemented though. If food rations from one harvest ran out some groups would be forced to fast for weeks at a time. This often took place in the early spring as the rations would exhaust throughout the winter, leaving the residents to fast until the blossoming of springs when there were foods available to be foraged and to be planted. Here we see intermittent fasting being utilized for survival, but for many of our ancestors there were spiritual reasons for fasting as well. Giving up something as precious as food was seen as a fitting sacrifice for the gods and deities. Also the heightened state of awareness that fasting induces was ideal for trying to commune with the gods. We see here a great wealth of human potential found in an intermittent fasting routine.

Even the influential Greek and Roman cultures advocated for an intermittent fasting routine. There are surviving writings and records of these cultures experiences with fasting. Hippocrates, thought to be the father of modern day medicine, wrote extensively on the benefits of fasting. He promoted the idea that fasting was key in living a long and healthy life. Hippocrates and the culture at the time found inspiration in nature when approaching medicine. Seeing that animals would not eat when they were ill, Hippocrates assumed that a sick body benefits form restricted caloric intake. Modern science has since confirmed this notion.

Paracelsus, who has been another influential presence in the modern world of medicine, also advocated fasting practices, stating, "Fasting is the greatest remedy of the physician within." Here he is referring to the natural ability for the body to heal itself through intermittent fasting practices. The positive effects of intermittent fasting on organ function have been proven by modern science. The idea that our bodies can be so self-sustaining is a concept that modern medicine has also struggled with. All the quick fix pills and diet fads have imposed the notion that we must act as an outside source to heal our bodies. We sell our bodies short with these ideas. Our bodies are capable of so much amazing potential why wouldn't they have healing mechanisms built in?

The Greek and Roman concepts of medicine are the foundation of modern medicine. Although today we put much less emphasis on the power of nature and the healing abilities our body is equipped with. There is no real reason for the advent of synthetic medicines except to optimize profits for large companies. These companies have monopolized the medicine industry making it very difficult for alternative medicines and natural therapies to be accessed by the majority of people. Plants cannot be patented, so these companies spend millions on synthetic chemicals that are able to mock the natural medicine's ability to combat disease. But at what cost ? The negative effects of unnatural medicines have been documented countless numbers of time through shared experiences from patients, adverse side effects and even contemporary studies. These detrimental medical practices are now the standard, all at the expense of the patient.

We see that the history of fasting is polarized by centuries of effective use embedded into human lifestyle versus only a few dozen decades worth of faulty science and questionable marketing tactics. We need to break these cycles, and in fact alter history.

Chapter 2: The Science of Fasting

We have found that fasting has history on its side in its battle for valid recognition. Our ancestors and some of the greatest thinkers known to man advocate for it But what does science have to say about the ancient practice? In recent decades solid evidence has been found to support claims of fasting's transformative powers. This has led to its popularity in fitness and health communities, while simultaneously being consistently upheld in spiritual communities as means of communing with the unknown. Even a short internet search with show that intermittent fasting is gaining momentum as a legitimate practice that is safe and effective.

It may seem simple to most people that intermittent fasting can lead to weight loss. Eat less food, gain less weight. But it is not quite as simple as this. There is an entire complex reaction our body has to a restricted calorie diet. The effects are unlike any other bodily function, affecting all parts of the body and mind. But practice must be taken seriously. You cannot expect to simply not eat and have the results you desire. You need to respect your body and the food you put into it. Let's take a look at the science and realize the incredible effects that fasting may yield. Below we will discuss the major organs and how they are effected by an intermittent fasting practice.

The Liver

The liver acts as the filtration system of the body. When the liver is not functioning properly any toxins or other unwanted compounds get stuck inside the body, causing all kinds of problems. The liver also produces bile. Bile is used to help aid in digestion while food is in the intestines. If the bile we produce is low quality then we cannot properly digest our foods.

When we are fasting the restriction of calories allows our liver some extra time to rest and rejuvenate. Without toxins from foods to filter the liver can efficiently relax and repair. Also while the liver is resting it is able to produce proteins that regulate its own function, allowing for optimal reparations. We see here that intermittent fasting helps the liver use its inherent abilities to heal itself and in turn perform its duties to heal the body.

The Heart

The heart's most important function is the regulation of blood flow. Nutrients are carried throughout the body in the blood stream, so without the hearth we cannot get the vitamins and minerals sufficient to operate our body. The heart is the most vital organ that acts autonomously, and heart disease is one of the leading factors of death in the western world. Intermittent fasting has been linked to reduce the effects of heart disease by allowing the heart to repair any damages. This resetting effect allows the heart to start anew and better heal itself.

The Brain

The mysterious human brain is the commander of all of our bodily functions. Our body sends signals to the brain to carry out other actions that are needed. While these reactions in the brain are subtle and not readily noticed when they take place, they are still greatly affected by intermittent fasting.

Since the brain is the epicenter of our entire being, emotional states, stress and overall health are regulated here by hormone production. Intermittent fasting acts directly on hormone regulation. When our bodies are deprived of food its response is similar to a defense mechanism, releasing hormones similar to the fight or flight response. The brain also responds by reducing metabolic rates to conserve energy and calories. If there are no immediate sources of energy form recently ingested food, the brain will signal the body to start burning fat reserves. This action paired with a healthy diet is the safest and most efficient way to burn fat and maintain a healthy weight.

Other Positive Results

Scientific evidence shows just what our ancestors had known; intermittent fasting is crucial in assisting our body's natural healing abilities. This being no small task for any diet, it is also simple and free. The major organs are not the only parts of our body that benefit from this practice, there are even more positive actions that accompany a fasting practice in our daily lives. Here are some examples of intermittent fasting's amazing results;

- Benefits growth hormone secretion. Similar effects may be reached through use of supplements, for example HGH, but the safety of these supplements is up for debate. Also, wouldn't a proven safe and natural regulation of growth hormones be more attractive?

- Assists the body with energy production by helping with the creation of mitochondria. These are the energy sources inside of all of our cells. Extra energy will help with stamina during exercise routines, other activities that require physical assertion.

- Calorie restricted diets leave the body no choice but to burn fat reserves for energy. Fat cells are known to be cleaner energy than carbohydrates and sugars. This will greatly reduce the release of free radicals which are linked to cancer due to the oxidation of cell walls.

- Intermittent fasting greatly reduces inflammation. Inflammation damages cells and leads to immune diseases and other problematic diseases. Intermittent fasting helps tocare for damaged cells when ketones are released through the burning of fat cells. Ketones help to

fight inflammatory problems. We will discuss ketosis in
detail in a later chapter.

-   Fasting may also prevent the body from becoming
    intolerant to insulin. Insulin intolerance may cause
    insulin to be over produced or sometimes not produce at
    all, which can lead to diabetic symptoms.

We find that the many benefits of intermittent fasting cannot be
ignored. Not only acting as a safe means to lose weight, the
practice also assists body to use its natural abilities to heal itself.
These are incredible benefits in a world that relies so heavily on
synthetic medicines and frequent doctor visits.

Misconceptions

There are many misconceptions about intermittent fasting as
well. This can be troublesome as you try and weed out good
information from bad information on the internet. Be careful
who you listen to and as always, do what works for you, not what
everybody else is doing. Below are some common
misconceptions pertaining to intermittent fasting.

Fasting slows down the metabolism
While your body will make the necessary adjustments to meal
patterns that are disrupted during intermittent fasting, it does
not 'slow' your metabolism. The metabolism is only in danger if
you manage to burn all your fat reserves, this is dangerous and
not recommended. While fasting we are striving to burn stored

fat reserves, but burning all of the fat is not something we are trying to do on purpose, nor is it something you can safely accomplish without detrimental reactions from your body.

People who fast can eat unhealthily
Some people believe that if you have an intermittent fasting routine then you are able to eat whatever you like whenever you want. There is no truth behind this notion. Your body requires high quality proteins, vitamins and minerals. Your may be able to live off of pizza, but you may not feel healthy or have energy. To maintain a healthful life our bodies need a variety of colorful foods. This variety will ensure our balanced and thriving state.

Fasting is just starving yourself
This is a popular standpoint for those who are against intermittent fasting. TO be starved is to burn all of your fat reserves, this is not easily done before becoming ill or losing consciousness. Also a proper fast is the intentional restricting of calories versus starving which is not a voluntary choice. We can be assured that we will not starve ourselves if we practice our intermittent fasting routine responsibly.

Fasting works for all people
While fasting is considered one of the safest means to lose weight and rebuild our relationship with food, it is not effective for everybody. People with any major disease should consult their physician before starting a fasting routine, especially those with diabetes. Although there are many shard experiences of

fasting's benefits, it is always best to listen to your body. Not one lifestyle change is going to work for absolutely everyone.

Fasting can lead to muscle loss
This is a very common misconception. While fasting can lead to increased fat loss, your muscles are not in danger of disappearing. While in extreme cases of starvation muscle loss is seen, it will not be something to worry about when practicing a safe intermittent fasting practice.

We find with the simple basics of intermittent fasting that there is a world of positive and negative opinions. This is to be expected toward a practice that can effectively heal the body for free. This may be too good to be true for many, but the human body is mysterious and even science knows very little of its amazing potential. We are hopeful that science will catch up with our distant ancestors and their views of the healing capabilities of the body.

While the history and science of this incredible practice are important as we continue the journey, we must also take into consideration our environment. Are we constantly stressed? Do we feel balanced in other aspects of our life beside our body? Mental health plays a huge role in the transformative effects of intermittent fasting as well. Not to mention the actual things you put into your body. All these aspects of living play an integral role in the transformative effects we strive to induce with this book.

Now that we have a firm grasp of the science and history of intermittent fasting we can venture in to the distinct techniques and styles that fasting has to offer.

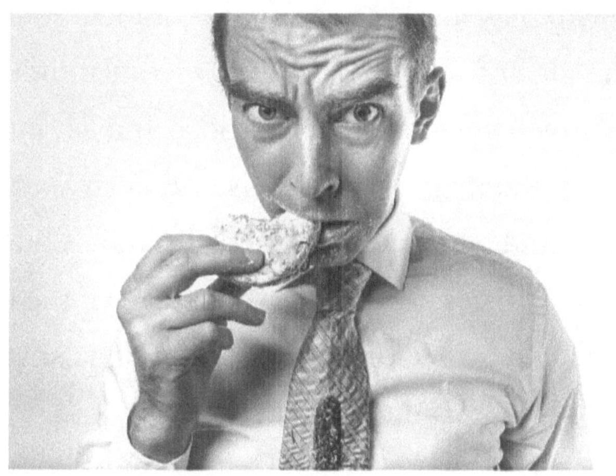

(Man eating slice of bread)

Chapter 3: Intermittent Fasting Techniques

Continuing our transformative journey, we need to take into consideration which intermittent fasting technique we wish to implement. Picture your desired life and think about your busy schedule, these will play a role in the choice of technique you choose. With the idea of weight loss heavy on our minds we need to consider how much weight we wish to lose and set individual goals for ourselves. Keep all of your goals and desires at the forefront of your mind when choosing a technique. Choose a technique that you feel comfortable with instead of the more challenging ones. Listen to your body and don't be ashamed if these techniques seem intimidating at first.

We have seen that intermittent fasting is rooted in spiritual practices. While these practices are no the focus of this book, you can easily fit your religious practices in with the following techniques. This chapter will define popular intermittent fasting methods in popular culture. There seem to be endless variations on an intermittent fasting practice, the techniques listed below are great starting points for beginners on the intermittent fasting path. You may wish customize your routine as it evolves over the course of months or years. With this evolution there will be an abundance of changes, physical and mental, some beginners find it beneficial to keep track of these experiences in a notebook. Developing awareness and mindfulness towards our bodies is key in getting the full benefits of fasting. By keeping track of our experiences we can organize our awareness and better anticipate our body's reactions to the restricted calorie days.

The techniques below are the most commonly practiced in the western world today. They are advocated by fitness and health experts alike as follows:

- The 5:2 technique
- The 16:8 technique
- The alternating day technique
- The eat stop eat technique
- The warrior technique
- The spontaneous technique
- OMAD or one meal a day

We will also look at ways to customize and alter these intermittent fasting techniques so that you may better fit them into your life. Being able to customize a practice is key to rebuilding our relationships with our bodies. We do not want to force ourselves into a routine that we do not enjoy. Feel free to alter and customize the techniques below for your needs. There will be some examples of alteration techniques after we explore the popular intermittent fasting styles.

The 5:2 Technique

Overview:
- 5 days of eating your typical diet
- 2 days of restricted calorie intake, less than 500

The 5:2 technique is great for people who are testing the waters with intermittent fasting. While many people wouldn't consider this a fast as much as a diet, it is popular among beginners and people with dietary allergies who want to test out an intermittent fasting practice. This method requires the practitioner to eat their typical diet for five days, and the remaining two days of the week will be the 'fasted' days, with a calorie restriction of less than 500 calories. As a customization technique you can alter the amount of caloric intake, add one to two hundred calories if it makes you more comfortable.

For this technique you choose your fasted days beforehand to prepare for the week. Once these days are chosen you can go about your business as usual. This casual method is great for easing into the intermittent fasting lifestyle as it does not require any intensive dry fasting or drastic lifestyle changes.

The 16:8 Technique

Overview:

- 16 hours without caloric intake
- 8 hour food intake timeframe
- Eat as much as you like during intake timeframe

This technique is quite popular among for people who have a little experience with fasting. This method asks of you to adhere to a sixteen hour fast, allowing for an eight hour window to eat. Sixteen hours may seem like forever, but consider the fact that you will more than likely be sleeping for half of that time.

For an example, you may awake after eight hours of sleeping, then refrain from caloric intake for eight hours, then eat whatever you like for the following eight hours. During the intake window you are allowed to eat whatever you want, but make healthy choices when you are choosing foods.

Alternating Day Technique

Overview:
-   Restrict calories every other day
-   Eat your typical diet on the other days

This method is self-explanatory with its title, you will be restricting calories every other day. This technique is ideal for beginners as it allows for simple alteration and customization. The fasted days can be zero calorie days or days restricted to a limited amount of calories. With this technique many people choose to alternate days and gradually lower caloric intake as they feel comfortable.

For an example you may start on Sunday and have a day of typical meals, Monday restrict calories, Tuesday have typical meals, Wednesday restrict calories and so on. This technique could be practiced safely for months at a time, but for beginners try one week and adjust accordingly.

Eat Stop Eat Technique

Overview:
- One fast day per week
- Typical diet on non-fast days

This method is great for a busy schedule. With the requirement of a zero calorie one day fast, it may be intimidating for beginners. You are allowed your usual diet for the non-fast days, but for the fasted day you can only ingest water, no calories whatsoever. These are the only rules, the timeframe you should be fasting should be at the least twenty-four hours.

For an example, you would elect your desired fast day beforehand and prepare for it accordingly. Go about your week as usual with the exception of this day. Once the fasted day arrives be sure to drink plenty of water and listen closely to your what your body is saying, restrict calorie intake to zero calories for twenty-four hours, and that's it. After this fasted day, you would continue on with your typical diet, until the next chosen fast day, which usually is planned for the following week. Some people may add two full fasted days to this technique if they so choose.

Warrior Technique

Overview:
  - Small portions of food during the day
  - Large, nutrient rich meal in the evening

This method is likened to a diet more than a fast similar to the 5:2 technique. While asking that you fast or restricted calories during daylight hours, you are able to have large meal in the evening. This technique also has the rule that you eat as healthy as possible, limiting sweets and processed foods. This technique is good for preparing for dry fasts, it keeps the intermittent fasting lifestyle at the forefront of the practitioner's mind.

Spontaneous Technique

Overview:

-   No strict rules

-   Skip meals when it is convenient

This method is great for busy schedules, you essentially just cut out meals whenever you desire or when it's convenient. There are no requirements or limitations, just do as you please making it a point to eliminate meals every once in a while. Not feeling hungry? Skip this meal. No time to prepare a meal? This is a great time to skip a meal. This method is great for those who adhere to a 'go with the flow' attitude towards living. Busy people may find themselves doing this without even thinking about the fact that they are not hungry. Many new parents will find themselves unintentionally missing meals, call it apart of your fast routine and move on! It should be noted here that mothers who are breastfeeding should not fast.

An example of this method is simple, you are having a busy week, there's no time to cook, so you just skip dinner and head to bed. This may seem too easy but it's a great way to break into the fasting lifestyle without compromising anything important in your life.

Alteration Techniques

With a basic knowledge of the popular intermittent fasting methods, we now need to have good ideas about how to customize these concepts to suit us as individuals. Most people are going to find their practice growing and changing. We need to see that fasting is able to fit itself into our routines as it wishes, and if we listen closely to our bodies we can work with our progress to find the most effective way to reach our desired goals through intermittent fasting practices.

This ability to alter our practice goes further to empower us to build a balanced relationship with our bodies and diets. By implementing distinct rules that are personalized and designed to help us, we can focus in on exactly what we need to accomplish with our goals and immerse ourselves in this transformative practice. Among the many different ideas for alteration and customization we have a general list of ideas including changing the length of fasting times, changing our diets to vegetarian or raw food diets, introducing sexercise and also altering the timing of fasting days to suit a busy work schedule.

The main purpose of the above techniques is to take control of our caloric intake and eating patterns. This seems like an blatant choice compared to the popular eating whenever and whatever, which runs rampant as a suitable lifestyle in our society. With this simple concept in mind, we can build an intermittent fasting routine that is personalized to our lives while also maintaining its effective results. When selecting to customize your routine consider all the variables. Am I actually ready to change my routine? Are the alterations I'm considering achievable? Do these customizations help me reach my chosen goals? We must keep the mantra in mind; No one practice is going to work for everyone. Customize your practice as you need, be patient and listen to your body. And don't be afraid to get creative and add your own customizations that may not be mentioned below.

Alteration Technique One: Lifestyle and Politics
The stereotype of the fitness fanatic is easily seen online, tanned and toned these people seem like they work out all day every day. This is not the majority and it's not the lifestyle everyone desires. When altering your routine take into consideration who you are. If you're not gym type of person, don't go to the gym. Essentially any other hobby can be a part of your newly found fasting routine, this is a point that cannot be stressed enough; intermittent fasting does not require you to change who you are or what you truly enjoy. If you like to paint then include painting on your fasting days to fill time that would normally be spent on cooking and cleaning. If you care for the environment include fasting in your convictions, less consumption means less waste. Include your passions into your routine and see them both as beneficial and healthy means of living.

Alteration Technique Two: Meal Timing

Many online resources claim that meal timing should be strictly adhered to, so if you're choosing to have a large meal in the evening, then your routine should reflect that consistently. This being said, you get to choose when your meal time is. With the warrior technique, which requires one large meal per day, you get to choose when the meal is. This can be applied to all the techniques, choose your meal time to suit your needs, not just based upon what others choose to do online. If you need to change your meal times in the midst of your set practice, do so gradually and with great care since your body will be accustom to having food at certain time.

Alteration Technique Three: Food Choices

If you feel that your diet is unhealthy and you desperately need to change it, you are not alone. Many people find themselves drawn to intermittent fasting to assist them in changing their food choices. These habits can seem impossible to change, but they certainly are not. When beginning an intermittent fasting routine, analyze your diet and see where you can improve the quality of your meals. IF and food choices work hand in hand, you can expect to keep eating fast food every day and get the full benefits from intermittent fasting, but you can use IF as a means to break habits and reevaluate your food choices. You're already changing your routine, might as well improve your food choices as well!

Many people take what they have learned through their fasting experiences and use their new routine to take on completely new food choices. Veganism, vegetarianism and raw food diets can be experimented with throughout your new routine. It is similar to the 'resetting' effect of organ function, only you are resetting your literal food choices. Try plant based foods only on certain days, or even for weeks at a time, or choose to eat only raw foods during intake windows. There are many diets to choose from, do your research and find what fits into your lifestyle.

Here we need to also address extreme cases of a bad diet. If you are overweight and have had unhealthy eating habits for many years, you may need to ease into your new routine and dietary choices. Gradually cut back on junk foods instead of going cold turkey. It is also recommended that you consult your physician to be extra safe when adopting new dietary practices.

Alteration Technique Four: Fasting Days
Most intermittent fasting plans will have strict guidelines for fasting days, but as you acclimate to the new routine you can change the fasting days to suit your schedule. Fasting days do not always have to be on Mondays, nor do they need to be consecutive if you are fasting multiple days in a week. Let your schedule decide your fasting days, plan it around menstrual cycles, or take a page from the spontaneous technique and randomly select days to fast.

Many choose to maintain patterns when intermittent fasting, and this is recommended to easily keep track and allow the body to settle into rest periods. But life changes suddenly, there is no shame in having to break a consistent pattern to allow a busy week to run more smoothly. Be open minded and aware when planning your fasts.

Alteration Technique Five: Intake Windows

As you examine the various techniques you see that one of the main differences is the timing and cycles of chosen fast days and intake times. The intake window is designed to allow plenty of time to eat while allowing ample time for the organ functions to rest and repair. While the intake windows are less customizable than the other aspects of intermittent fasting, you can still choose time frames that are fitting for your personal needs. Some may opt to shorten intake windows, while others may need a slightly longer intake window to sync up with busy schedules or ease into the practice safely.

With all the different variations that can be used to personalize an intermittent fasting routine, it is rare that the practice can't be fit into one's life. Be open minded and listen to what your body is saying. Do not be afraid to cancel a fast if you are uncomfortable with the experience, always put your safety first and don't hesitate to have a bite to eat if you feel light headed or dizzy.

The popular techniques of intermittent fasting are popular for a reason, the fitness gurus and online communities advocate for these techniques because they work. These people are happy to offer their experiences and advice online, creating a space that validates IF as a safe and effective means of transforming one's life for the better. Now that we have a general idea of the practices and routines themselves, let's look at how weight loss is directly related an intermittent fasting routine.

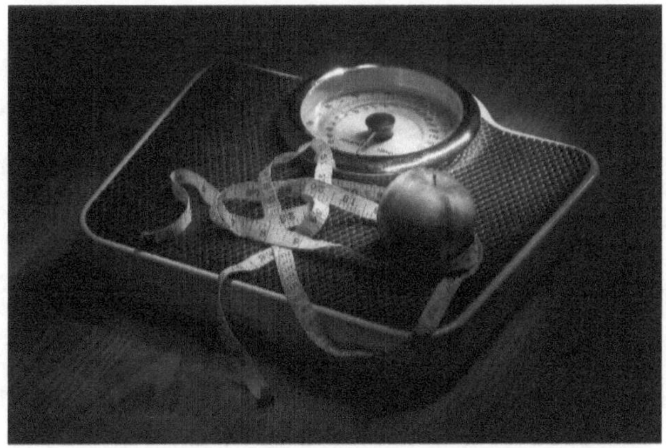

(Balance and an apple)

Chapter 4: What is Ketosis?

Ketosis and ketogenic states have been a very popular topic of conversation in scientific and fitness communities. The state of ketosis is advocated by many people who practice an intermittent fasting routine, especially as a means to lose weight quickly. Intermittent fasting and ketosis are closely related, in fact ketosis is induced through restricted calorie diets. But what exactly is ketosis?

The ketogenic state is a natural process that occurs in the body. As we have discussed, fat reserves are the go to alternative for energy when our bodies have no quick energy to burn. When our fat reserves are burned in this way ketones are released into the blood. This is ketosis. Although, this metabolic state is not always favorable. When ketones are released the blood gets very acidic, this can lead to detrimental levels of acidity in the blood. When blood levels are too acidic the state of ketoacidosis can occur. This is very dangerous and can lead to death.

Usually hormones such as insulin help to regulate ketone levels, stopping them from becoming too high. When you enter a state of ketoacidosis there is nothing your body can do to stop the overwhelming amount of ketones that are being produced. This causes many problems for people with diabetes. Since diabetic symptoms are heavily reliant on insulin production, diabetic patients are at a greater risk of inducing ketoacidosis.

Ketosis

For weight loss there is growing interest and conversation on the subject of ketosis and ketogenic diets. The ketogenic state that can be attained has been shown to produce great results, especially concerning weight loss. While a ketogenic diet is not necessary for an intermittent fasting routine, it is recommended that the science of ketosis and its relation to IF be recognized.

Ketosis is a naturally occurring metabolic process within the body. When our bodies burn stored fat cells instead of quick energy from recently ingested foods, ketones are produced and the ketogenic state is induced. Although it is popular in the current culture and many success stories are available online, the state of ketosis isn't always a positive thing. Depending on how the ketosis is induced and overall context of the situation, an unbalanced level of ketones in the blood is not desirable. If these levels reach numbers that are too high complications can occur. Typically hormones such as insulin regulate ketone levels, preventing them from becoming too high, but if your body isn't producing the needed amount of insulin the ketone levels can get out of control and become too high. This is where many diabetic may find that they are in an unwanted ketogenic state, their bodies not producing adequate insulin and not regulating the ketones. We will go into detail on diabetes and intermittent fasting in a later chapter.

Bodies that functions well will typically won't even produce ketones. Having a balanced diet with plenty of quick energy in the form of sugars and carbohydrates will allow the body to avoid a ketogenic state. We see here that ketosis is not unlike other survival mechanisms that are natural built into our bodies. IF there is no quick access to energy our bodies soon creates ketones and starts burning stored fat cells. Besides calorie restriction and perhaps an intensive exercise session, a ketogenic state will likely not be induced. The Ketogenic state is the link between intermittent fasting and effective weight loss, this state quite literally burns of our fat reserves.

Ketoacidosis

With all the success stories and research ketogenic diets may seem like the key to success when I comes to weight loss. But we need to keep in mind that inducing this state requires a serious attention to detail. If you intentionally induce a ketogenic state and your ketones levels get too high, you may experience ketoacidosis. This reaction to high ketone levels in the blood turn the blood very acidic, this can cause comas or in some extreme cases even death. It is recommended that if a ketogenic diet is practiced that you test your urine or blood using a test kit. Careless fasting practices can lead to ketoacidosis, other common culprits include dehydration and alcoholism. If you have had issues with insulin production, thyroid over activity or alcoholism, it is best to consult your physician before attempting a ketogenic diet.

A body that functions on a healthy level will not typically create ketones. With plenty of quick energy to burn and ample fat reserves a body will run efficiently without any problem of inducing ketoacidosis. For those who are practicing an intermittent fasting practice we need to be very aware of the ketogenic state and make sure not to induce ketoacidosis unintentionally. For those that are inducing it intentionally, they need to be very experienced and aware of their bodies.

Intermittent Fasting and Diabetes

There needs to be a special section on the relationship between diabetes and fasting since they are both closely linked to the ketogenic state. Diabetes is a very common disease and some studies have shown that fasting may decrease the risk of developing diabetes for those who have not been diagnosed. Many feel that diabetes should not be paired with intermittent fasting while others feel that they can be practiced safely together. This is going to vary individual to individual and should always involve a physician's opinion on the safety. Let's discuss the basic of diabetes and diabetic symptoms.

The symptoms of diabetes can be subtle, slowly getting worse and worse with time whether the individual knows they have it or not. Many people suffer from acute diabetic symptoms, known as prediabetes or borderline diabetes, these people do not even realize they have these symptoms. Diabetes is a commonly diagnosed disease where your blood sugar levels can get too high. We see here the close link between ketosis and diabetes. The sugars we get from foods are needed for energy to do anything, from day to day tasks to intensive exercises. Insulin is produced and helps these sugars find their way to our body's cells. If your body is having trouble creating insulin, you could have diabetes. If the insulin isn't effectively regulating the sugars, blood-sugar ratios can be off balance causing diabetic-like symptoms.

There are two types of diabetes, as well as borderline or prediabetes, which usually becomes a full diabetic issue in years to come. Let's discuss these types and differences between them.

Type 1 Diabetes

This type of diabetic disease is not as common as its counterpart. Having Type 1 Diabetes means that your body does not produce insulin at all. This requires insulin shots to help regulate sugars in the bloodstream.

Type 2 Diabetes

Your body not producing sufficient amounts of insulin or not being able to use the insulin that is produced successfully characterizes the more common type of diabetic disease, Type 2 Diabetes.

Prediabetes

If your blood sugar levels are higher than average but not high enough to be considered diabetic, you may have prediabetes. This will need to be monitored as it puts you at risk for Type 2 diabetes in the future.

Blood tests can verify if you have diabetes. While it is a serious disease, many people lead fulfilling lives with diabetes. We are able to control our diabetic symptoms with exercise and specific meal plans. Monitoring your blood sugar levels is a common practice as well. While taking insulin shots is a common perception of people with diabetes, these measures are not usually the first step of management for Type 2 sufferers. Prescription pharmaceuticals and shifting diet and lifestyle to healthier practices can also help manage diabetic symptoms. With this in mind, let's take a look at what an ideal diet would look like to manage diabetes.

Diabetes Diet

Changes in diet are common means to combat diabetic symptoms. It is often the first step to take if one is diagnosed with prediabetes. Simple changes in meal plans have a great effect on organ function as we have previously discussed. This includes the pancreas, where insulin production begins. Naturally, change in diet and the relationship with food are effective ways to manage and regulate blood sugar levels. Examining your diet and making the necessary changes is crucial for natural management of blood sugar levels.

Diets designed specifically to combat diabetic symptoms are simple; we need to intake moderate amounts of healthy food and make sure to keep a strict pattern of meal times. This means eating at the same time every day and typically at favorable times of the day, not in the middle of the night when our digestive systems prefer to rest. As with any healthy diet, we need nutrient-rich foods that are not processed. Low-fat ingredients and foods that are low in calorie count are ideal as well. The diet emphasizes fresh fruits, vegetables, whole grains, and legumes. Low in fat dairy ingredients are accepted as well but many people exclude these products as well.

The ideal diet for diabetes is a balanced diet for anyone. It's as simple as keeping your diet fresh and wholesome and giving up sugary snacks especially soda and candies. Diets of this nature are key for losing weight as well. Studies have shown that weight loss can also help with the management of diabetic symptoms, making it much easier to monitor and control blood sugar levels.

Carbohydrates

Our main source of sugars for energy, in the form of glucose, comes from carbohydrates. Carbs break down and transform into glucose for our body to use as quick energy. This means carbs have the greatest role to play in the blood-sugar levels. People with diabetes must watch carefully how many carbohydrates they consume to help balance out the blood-sugar levels and if they take insulin, they will need to adjust the dosage accordingly.

With help from a dietician, many people with diabetes educate themselves on how to efficiently read food labels and track their carbohydrate intake. This is a mild inconvenience that is crucial to the diabetic diet. Always consult your physician or dietician when adjusting insulin dosage.

Glycemic Index

Some people use the glycemic index to measure and choose foods, in particular, carbohydrates. This index is a system that ranks various foods depending on their effects on the sugar levels in the blood. The glycemic index is used on a scale of 1-100. There are three main categorizations for GI, they are as follows; Low, Moderate, and High. These groups are pretty self-explanatory. A glycemic index that is considered low is a score of 55 or less, a moderate index is 56 -69, and the high index is 70 or more. Lower indexed carbs are metabolized slower and cause a much more gradual rise in blood sugar levels and in turn slower rise in insulin levels. Higher indexed carbs metabolize more quickly and cause more insulin to be produced, thus being more difficult to regulate.

An average American day of meals has a glycemic index of 50-60. For people with diabetes, it can be safe to assume that a much lower GI is ideal, around 45 for an entire day. This number can even be lower if one chooses to be extra careful with their carb intake. Studies have shown that from around the world the lowest glycemic indexes on average are 40-45. There are numerous health benefits linked to these low indexes as well, including a lowered risk of heart disease and lowered risk of developing diabetes.

Below we will include a diabetes diet plan. It is safe to say that this plan is also a balanced diet for anyone, even without diabetes.

Basic Diabetes Diet Plan

When developing a plan to alter your diet to assist in the regulation of blood sugar levels we need to take great care and attention to detail. Many who are diagnosed with diabetic symptoms are referred to a dietician to help prepare and initiate a new meal plan. Below we will give a basic outline of how a diabetes diet plan would be practiced.

Diabetes diets require three moderately sized meals each day at the usual meal times. Breakfast, lunch, and dinner times being an ideal pattern to adopt. These meals will be small to medium in size so we need to make the portions count by choosing nutrient-dense ingredients and filling foods such as whole grains and healthy fats. Each meal should be balanced with a nice variety of foods. The diabetic diet-shopping list would look like this;

- Healthy Carbohydrates such as fruits, vegetables, whole grains, and beans. Avoid processed foods with added sugars and fats.
- Fish, such as tuna and salmon. Avoid fish high in mercury.
- Fiber-filled foods such as vegetables, fruits, and nuts.

- Healthy fats from avocados, olive oil, and nuts.

There are also foods that need to be avoided on a diabetes diet. Foods that are notorious for increasing the risk of heart disease or hardening arteries should be completely avoided. These foods contain;

- Unhealthy fats found in beef, butter, margarine, and processed snacks.
- Cholesterol found in dairy and eggs.

The less processed the ingredient the less likely it is going to contain these detrimental compounds. It is also recommended that the adherents of this diet ingest less than 2,500 mg of sodium per day. This number varies greatly person to person so consult your physician for details on this amount as it pertains to you.

When putting together meal plans specifically for diabetes, the main focus is to include more vegetables. But we need to balance the brightly colored, nutrient-rich ingredients with tan starches, and lean sources of protein. As a general guideline this is ideal;

- Half or more of your portion of food should consist of vegetables like carrots, kale, or tomatoes.

- One-fourth of your portion should consist of lean proteins like fish or chicken.
- One-eighth of your portion should consist of whole grains like brown rice or quinoa.
- One-eighth of your portion should consist of starchy vegetables like peas or potatoes.
- For small snacks in between meals choose a serving of healthy fats like an avocado or a single serving of fruit.
- For drinks choose unsweetened ones and plenty of water. Avoid fruit juices for their concentrated sugar content. Coffee and teas are great in between meals, but of course, unsweetened.

This general guide is perfect for a diabetes diet and since the disease is so dangerous, this structure should be adhered to with great attention to detail. There are other aspects of this lifestyle that need extra attention as well.

We see that the ketogenic state can have its benefits, but there are also great dangers involved when approaching this practice. When deciding if inducing ketosis for health reasons is right for your practice you must be one hundred percent sure that you do not have diabetes or diabetic symptoms. If you do have these problems you must work closely with your physician for any type of fast, especially one that may induce ketosis intentionally.

While many people may try and tell you that no one should induce ketosis, this is not their decision to make. This is your practice and you call the shots. Make intelligent decisions and listen to your body as you approach more intensive fasting practices. These practices are to be respected and held in high regard. For beginners these methods are not recommended, but as you progress you may be looking for more challenging limitations on your fasting routine. Always remember to be cautious and really take the time to contemplate whether or not these more challenging routines are for you.

Ketosis may not be on everyone's mind when they first approach an intermittent fasting routine, but being educated on this naturally occurring state is a must for any serious intermittent fasting practice. If ketosis is unintentionally induced there are telling signs to look out for. As always if you feel any discomfort you must end your fast and find out why. Ketoacidosis also will make your breath and body odor have a very acidic smell. This is the main signal that our blood's ketone levels are too high.

Educating yourself on the dangers of intermittent fasting is just as important as learning the benefits and positive attributes of the practice. Ketosis and the ketogenic state is a perfect example of how something beneficial and naturally occurring in the body can be life threatening. Do not scrimp on your education of intermittent fasting practices and of course, listen to your body as much as possible, it is designed to heal and care for itself.

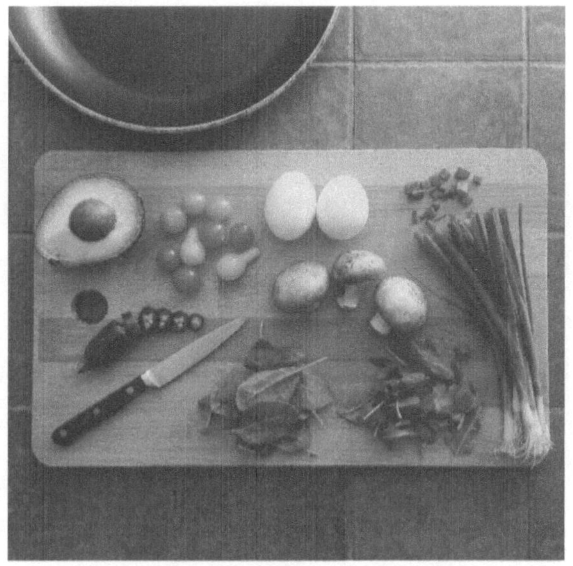

(Ketogenic raw ingredients)

Chapter 5: The Intermittent Fasting Diet

We have examined many crucial points of intermittent fasting, but we must also examine our diets and food choices. An intermittent fasting practice does not require physical activity or scientific knowledge of our body, but it helps to be familiar with these ideas. Even if you leave the exercise and science behind, the reactions are still occurring in your body. Calorie restrictions are the very basic premise of fasting and for most people this will mean changing your diet, sometimes very dramatically.

The following chapter will be comprised of a detailed look at what kind of diet is ideal for an intermittent fasting practice. This practice isn't as simple as cutting out all unhealthy food, we must take time to rebuild a healthy relationship with our bodies and diets. You should be paying close attention to food labels and nutritional ingredients. Consider where your food is grown and sourced. Are your foods processed or filled with synthetic preservatives? Paying close attention to these details will go a long way in initiating your transformative new lifestyle.

Take a look at what you have eaten in the past week. Would you consider these meals healthy? How processed are these ingredients? Were you eating because you were hungry or because you are supposed to? Where are these foods sourced?

Were there any raw foods? Did you prepare and cook these foods?

The examination of our typical diet will allow us to gain an outsider's perspective on our own food choices. We can see our food intake and consider the needed changes that we must begin. Be meticulous and judgmental when you examine your diet, what changes need to be made? Will the new diet cost more money? Organize these concepts and keep them at the front of your mind, this is a great first step to altering our food choices for the better.

Think about your next trip to the grocery store. When we are ready to begin a fast it is recommended that we make any necessary dietary changes as well. It is good advice to begin on a more nutritious diet before we begin our fasting routine, especially if you consider you diet to be extremely unhealthy. Eliminate junk food an over processed foods if they are abundant in your diet. Especially if you are overweight it is recommended to improve your diet before beginning an intermittent fasting routine.

Diet and Food

For unnecessary weight gain and overall bad health there are many culprits. The food supply being greatly genetically modified and grown in soil that lacks a balanced nutrient content has been a controversial environmental issue for decades. When we notice that most of our foods found in large super markets are overly processed and full of synthetic chemical we may quickly become discouraged at the hopes of attaining a healthy diet. It may seem unavoidable to eat overly processed ingredients, but there are measures that can be taken to improve our diets, from sourcing our food from local farms, to choosing a broader variety of foods as a whole.

Searching for foods that are grown locally will allow you to have more control over the quality of the ingredients you ingest. Locally grown vegetables and fruits, locally raised meat and fresh grains are often produced without using pesticides. When we source our foods locally we also promote community and local economy. These foods are more nutrient rich and typically taste better as well.

Not all regions have access to local produce and ingredients, this can be challenging for many people when trying to make healthful food choices. If local food is not available you can still make better choices at the super market. Buy fresh produce like veggies and fruits, avoid processed snacks and purchase organic ingredients when feasible. Organically grown food may be more expensive but these products worth it, especially with foods that are famous for being genetically modified such as potatoes, soy, corn and rice.

We now know there are plenty of variables that affect our health. Aspects like exercise and food choices, as well intangible factors like stress and correct organ function. All these concepts are distinctly improved by intermittent fasting. We start to see a pattern in the overall science of fasting and the areas of life it has influence upon. When we see this pattern form we can visualize a healthy lifestyle that is self-sustainable and easy to implement, which will certainly lead to a healthy weight and appearance. These relationships cannot be ignored if we wish to understand how these practices work to not only shed unwanted weight, but also form a positive and confident self-image.

Foods for Intermittent Fasting

There are thousands of different diets and food fads to be found online, this can make it hard to know what is a truly healthy diet. Many of these fads are simply concepts to eliminate troublesome foods rather than create a balanced diet. Many of these diets are not even based in science. These diets are rarely based on balanced nutritional meal. These fads also usually only focus on the importance of certain foods, rather than offering other effective ideas like exercising or having a positive attitude.

Intermittent fasting is not a fad, we have seen the history and modern science, when applied properly to your life, fasting is safe and natural than other diets that only require the abstinence from certain foods. Intermittent fasting is so easily approached since it does not require the complete abandonment of your favorite foods completely, only during small windows of time. As you consider how to improve your diet, consider the fact that you are not being asked to completely uproot your entire routine. There is still value in the indulgence of our favorite foods, you should not force yourself into an unenjoyable situation. Cheat days come in handy for this, they act to break up the patterns and give a reward for your discipline. Do not use cheat days as an excuse to overindulge, this defeats the purpose of our intermittent fasting practice altogether.

It is safe to say that suitable foods for an effective intermittent fasting routine are not processed or synthetic. Foods that are natural and sourced as locally as possible will be ideal for any fasting routine, but this may not be feasible for everyone. Do not be discouraged and do the best you can to use nutrient rich foods. The following lost will be some ingredients that are perfect for improving your diet and building a balanced relationship with food. This list definitely does not cover all the great foods out there, but it is designed to contain easily accessible foods that are among the most popular in health circles.

If the following foods are not included in your diet it is recommended that you make it a point to include them before or during your new intermittent fasting practice. This is great way to rebuild your relationship with food, learn what foods you can source locally. Find out how these foods help your body and gain a general knowledge of the foods in your diet. Learn to appreciate the flavors and the foods themselves as you introduce them into your diet.

This list is in alphabetical order for easy reference.

Almonds

Nuts are packed full when it comes to nutrient density. Almonds are among some of the more nutritious nuts, these small snacks are packed with protein, copper, vitamin E, and magnesium. Although these snacks are full of calories so be cautious on calorie-restricted days.

Blue Berries and Black Berries

Blueberries and blackberries are among the most popular in health circles. They are very rich in antioxidants, and add a nice acidity and sweetness on low calorie days.

Broccoli

Broccoli is famous for being hated by some, but this veggie is full of vitamin K and vitamin C, while also boasting a variety of minerals.

Beans

Black beans, garbanzo and kidney beans all contain an ample amount of protein, making them popular in plant-based diets.

Carrots

Carrots contain vitamins and minerals, as well as having lots of fiber and antioxidants. Once they are cooked or steamed they sweeten adding a nice contrast to savory dishes like stir fry and soups. Not to mention they add a nice flavor and brightness to salads.

Cauliflower

Often overlooked due to its similar looking counterpart, broccoli. Cauliflower is incredibly nutrient dense containing high amounts of vitamin C and vitamin K. Its fiber content is notable as well. There are some very creative uses for cauliflower as its popularity grows, including cauliflower pizzas and steaks. Also adds some needed nutrients to salads.

Chocolate

Aside from overly processed name brand chocolate bars, chocolate in an organic state is actually quite nutritious. Fiber, iron, antioxidants and many other valuable nutrients are pack into bitter dark chocolate. Find some sustainably sourced chocolate at a specialty store and make hot coco, or nibble as a snack in between meals.

Dates

This is one of the sweeter foods on our list, and it gets a place for good reason. For a sweet snack not many other foods have the vitamin and antioxidant content that dates have. They are considered a super food and are perfect for a healthy sweet snack or used in appetizers paired with cheeses.

Dandelion

These lovely flowers get an honorable mention for their vitamin C content and antioxidant value. Also the tea of these flowers and roots act as diuretic, which can help cleanse a body that has been maintaining a toxic diet for many years. Very low in caloric intake, it is great for restricted calorie days.

Eggplant

Vitamins, minerals and fiber make up this distinct food. We mentioned colorful foods are typically healthy and there aren't many foods that are so purple! Add to stir fry or gourmet recipes like eggplant Parmesan.

Flax Seed

A popular alternative to eggs in vegan baked goods, flax seed is rich in omega-3s and other fatty acids. Along with fiber and protein, this food is great for alternatives to wheat flours or expensive nuts. Add to salads, smoothies or find a bread recipe that relies on flax.

Fish

Of the variety of meat available to consumers, fish is going to be the go to option for weight loss and overall health. Much leaner than beef or pork, fish is considered healthier all around. Rich in iron, protein and minerals, fish such as salmon, halibut and tuna are among some of the most popular.

Garlic

Found in many recipes, garlic offers much in vitamins and minerals, while also helping regulate blood pressure. Garlic contains antibacterial properties as well, so naturally it finds itself as a part of cleanses and purifying raw diets.

Grapes

These tasty little snacks are not only a popular children's food, but has been proven to contain a distinct phytochemical named resveratrol. This phytochemical has been linked to prevent cancer growth and is popular among the supplement community. Even in its fermented form, wine, this food is considered healthy in small amounts.

Green Tea

Having only four calories per twelve ounce serving, green tea is great for calorie restricted days. Although containing caffeine, there are other chemicals that counteract the jittery effects of caffeine found in coffees. Great for calorie restricted mornings and needed antioxidants and minerals.

Grains

Whole grains such as rice, bulgur, corn and oats have a bit of protein and fiber, but also yield a large amount of carbohydrates which can be good for some quick energy to burn. Choose breads that are whole grain, preferably baked locally from fresh flours. Oatmeal, granola and a slice of toast in the morning are great small meals to begin a day.

Honey

Essentially containing no protein, fat or fiber, honey is a great alternative to table sugars and other sweeteners. Not to mention locally sourced honey has been proven to assist with allergic reactions, sore throats and boasts an impressive antioxidant content.

Kale

This leafy green has become popular over the years as an easy to grow, nutrient dense food. Small amounts of protein and tons of vitamins, one of the best sources of vitamin K, Kale is fibrous and perfect for smoothies or steamed for a savory side.

Lemon

You can get one third of your needed vitamin C from a quarter cup of lemon juice. Low caloric content and plenty of minerals, lemon juice also has antimicrobial compounds which make it ideal for cleanses and low calorie days. Drink straight cut with water, include in smoothies or use as main ingredient in other refreshing libation.

Lentils

Similar to beans, lentils provide and extraordinary amount of protein making it a popular staple in plant based diets. Ketogenic diets love lentils as well, plenty of fiber and a low carb count make them ideal. Add to soups or as an alternative to beans in any recipe.

Melons

Watermelon, honeydew, cantaloupe and a variety of other melons are great when you're in need of a sweet snack. A moderate level of calories means you need to watch melon on calorie restricted days, otherwise they are a great snack to get the vitamins and minerals needed. Eat sparingly as there is a high sugar content.

Mushrooms

Low calorie and low carb mushrooms offer soluble fiber, vitamins and minerals while containing no fiber or cholesterol. The distinct flavor and texture adds 'meatier' feeling to chilis and soups, making mushrooms desirable to vegan and vegetarian diets.

Onion

The pungent aroma and distinct flavor make onions a welcome addition to savory meals. With a very low calorie count they are ideal for low calorie days, without sacrificing flavor. Onions are known to have detoxifying affects as well. Add to any meal that needs a kick of flavor, or raw in salads.

Olive Oil

This fatty oil is not your friend on calorie restricted days, but during intake windows olive oil will provide you plenty of healthy fats and calories to burn as quick energy. Cook with olive oil instead of low quality vegetable oils or butters.

Potatoes

Root vegetables tend to be very filling with low calorie count, this makes them ideal for intake windows even if we are restricting calories. Also boasting high vitamin and mineral content, potatoes are versatile and nutritious. Bake or steam for a filling side dish.

Quinoa

This old world grain has seen a surge in popularity in the past decade. This is due mainly to its versatility as an alternative to rice or pasta, but with more protein. Also quinoa is more flavorful than its starchy alternatives. Replace rice with quinoa in any recipe to boost the protein content.

Rice

The most consumed food in the world, rice is readily available and cheap. Small amounts of protein and minerals. This grain is very low in calorie content making it a staple during an intermittent fasting diet. Rice is filling and versatile, add as a side with suitable seasoning, or mix with veggies for a stir fry.

Seeds

Chia seeds, flax seeds, sunflower seeds and an abundant array of many other types of seeds are some the most nutrient dense foods that are available. Packed with protein these foods are a perfect snack during intake windows, offering quick energy and a filling texture. Be careful on calorie restricted days since seeds are a high calorie food. Mix into salads or smoothies, or snack on them raw.

Spinach

A popular leafy green for good reason. Spinach offers plenty of fiber and vitamins, while keeping an incredibly low calorie count. Spinach has been over shadowed by kale in recent years, but still is a valuable addition to smoothies and salads. Replace lettuce with spinach in any recipe for added nutritional value.

Sweet Potato

Although not an actual potato, this root vegetable has more vitamin content than potatoes and also boast on of the highest potassium contents of any food. The calorie content is moderate, and sweet potatoes offer a healthy sweetness to many meals. Bake and use for savory dishes, get creative with sweet potato tacos.

Soy

There is some controversy regarding soy beans phytoestrogens, but little science has proven any extreme negative effects. Soy has become a staple in vegan and vegetarian diets for its excellent source of quality protein. Ingest raw as edamame, fermented as tofu or in soups.

Shellfish

Oysters, mussels, crab and shrimp offer healthy fats and omegas, while also being a low calorie source of protein. These foods can be a nice break from mundane foods, their distinct flavor and preparation is a nice escape form typical meals. Go out to a reputable seafood restaurant or if you have the skills, prepare at home steamed and lightly seasoned.

Tofu

Not to be redundant, but tofu gets another look even though it's mentioned in the soy category. Tofu is essentially fermented soy bean. It is full of protein and low in caloric intake. Not to mention its versatility, tofu will effectively take on any flavor you expose it to, making it great for plant based diets and a meat alternative. Sauté in a stir fry, or marinate and roast with root veggies.

Tomatoes

Tomatoes are rich in potassium and other vitamins and also boast a wide array of different varieties to choose from. The bright flavors are great added to salads or eaten on their own.

Venison

Of the many lean meats venison loin can be the best bang for your buck. Although not great for calorie restricted diets, it can be great for intake windows, especially similar patterns found in the warrior diet. Replace beef or pork with venison as needed.

This may not be a list of all the healthy ingredients in the world, but they are some of the most readily available and nutritious you can find. Use this list as a reference to find ingredients that are going to improve your diet. Notice that the list is comprised of colorful foods. It is safe to say that the more colorful your diet the better it is for you. Many vitamins and minerals are what give these foods their eye-popping colors.

Intermittent fasting Diets

With all the fad diets and popular trends in food it can be difficult to find a suitable one on the internet. Fads come and go, but there are diets that have been consistent throughout the decades. Many fads are loose variations on these diets, among them veganism and raw food diets. When you desire to improve your diet choose time tested dietary routines, ones based on balanced food choices or of valuable cultural significance. When you are deciding on a diet choose what will work for you. You can have vegetarian days sometimes and other times eat your typical meals. Maybe you want to have a raw food day each week. The possibilities are endless, but create a diet plan that you will be happy with.

Let's now explore the diets that are most suited to fit in with an intermittent fasting practice. The following list is designed to offer a nice variety of diets to choose from, all of the choices being great candidates for an intermittent fasting routine.

Raw Food

The guidelines for this diet are simple: only ingest raw foods. Some people seeking to practice this diet slowly introduce raw foods into their typical diet until they feel that they are comfortable with the completely raw diet. To reiterate; raw means uncooked, unprocessed ingredients. No preservation or added ingredients, but raw, fresh ingredients, maybe lightly seasoned.

This diet does require consistent access to fresh ingredients which may not be available for everyone. This diet is probably the toughest to maintain. With the least amount of ingredient options available, the raw diet consists mainly of nuts seeds, fruits of vegetables.

Since there is minimal cooking needed for this diet, many opt for smoothies or shakes to fill up quick during a busy schedule. Otherwise salads and snack style meals throughout the day comprise this diet.

Paleo

The paleo diet has seen a rise popularity in recent years, gaining the attention of fitness communities. This diet draws inspiration from diet that we believe our ancestors consumed in hunter-gatherer cultures. These cultures ate mostly raw foods that they had hunted or foraged for on the day of ingestion. This diet would include nuts, berries, meat or fish and herbs. Even modern studies have shown insight into these eras, suggesting that our ancestors were incredibly active and consumed mainly raw ingredients. The paleo diet is often misconceived as a meat only diet. While meat can be a major part of the diet, there is plenty evidence that suggests that plant-based foods would make up the majority of the diet.

We also see with hunter gatherer cultures that there may not have always been a successful hunt, resulting in days of lower

caloric intake for the large tribes. This was certainly
implemented in spiritual ways as well, fasting before important
celebrations or other holidays.

Paleo diets can be defined in many ways, but overall the
structure is maintained; mostly raw foods and fresh ingredients.
Preferably locally sourced or ethically sourced. Lean meats and
seafood, root vegetables, nuts, fruits and herbs.

We must also consider that during these times there was no
agriculture so many people adhering to a strict paleo diet would
exclude products of domestication or agriculture. These
products include dairy products, breads and any processed
foods of course.

Whole Thirty
The whole thirty diet has seen a rise in popularity as more
people have realized their gluten intolerances and other subtle
allergies. The whole thirty diet is a practice of identifying these
allergens and subsequently exclude them from your diet. You
will cut out common foods that are culprits for developing
allergies, then reintroduce them slowly and see if you have any
adverse reactions. If you discover that you have a slight allergy
to peanuts, for example, then you would exclude them from your
diet.

This diet asks that you cleanse for thirty days from common foods that people are allergic to. Peanuts, beans, grains, fish, dairy and soy are all common culprits for people's allergies. Exclude these foods for thirty days then slowly reintroduce them and take note of your body's reactions.

There are many foods that can be causing unfavorable reactions inside your body, so if you suspect another food that is causing trouble give it the thirty day treatment as well.

This diet is great for developing awareness of our bodies. We are essentially getting in tune with ourselves and learning what ingredients may be causing trouble. This will help us rebuild our relationship with our diets and food as a whole. This is great for our purposes in this book, intermittent fasting fits in well with the whole thirty diet.

Vegetarian Diets

Many cultures from around the world have adhered to a vegetarian diet. Plant based foods have a spiritual significance that many religions have practiced as well. These diets have grown in popularity in recent decades as many people see the factory farming industry to be unethical. The reliance on meat products has impacted the environment and our health in detrimental ways, being a leading cause of heart disease as well as pollution.

The requirements to adhere to a vegetarian diet are pretty easy. You only ingest plant based foods. Some vegetarians still consume dairy and eggs, but still stay away from meat products. This is closely related to the vegan diet, although vegans avoid all animal products.

A vegetarian diet is great for those who wish to change their diet dramatically but still enjoy hearty meals. The added fact that it's better for the environment is great as well. Vegetables, nuts fruits, whole grains, beans and soy products are staples of the vegetarian diet.

Vegan

The vegan diet is quite similar to the vegetarian diet, but it is much more strict. In a vegetarian diet you are able to eat eggs or dairy, for vegans all animal products are off limits. This means no milk, eggs, animal broths, cheese or honey. Any product that uses any animal ingredients is off limits. Here we see that veganism has a philosophy built in, they aim to rid the world of animal cruelty. While our purposes in this book are not concerned with animal rights, it is still good to touch on the diet itself. Vegetables, fruits, whole grains, nuts and soy products are crucial ingredients for a vegan diet.

Mediterranean

This diet is based in the diet that is eaten in the Mediterranean region. This region is well known for its celebratory dining and overall positive outlook on life. With this rich culture we also find a very healthy diet. Here we see that this culture has a healthy and balanced relationship with diet and food. Many ingredients are locally sourced and the people of the Mediterranean are walking examples of the success of this diet. Fruits, legumes, fish, vegetables and olive oil are integral for this diet.

Ketogenic

We have discussed ketosis and ketogenic states earlier in the book, but there is a diet that is used to safely induce ketosis in small amounts. Here we must reiterate the dangers of ketogenic states, you must be very careful when approaching this practice. Be sure to listen closely to your body and consult a physician for any in depth questions.

Ketogenic diets are typically very low in sugars and high in healthy fats and proteins. This helps to control caloric intake and better manage the ketones that are released into your bloodstream. Eggs, avocados, olive oil, fatty meats and fish rule this diet.

We need to again touch on the basics of ketosis. This is not a practice that is suitable for beginners, it can be very dangerous and you must treat it with respect and humility. Limiting your caloric intake even if you are still eating other foods will still induce a ketogenic state. Cutting out breads, rice, potatoes and other carb heavy foods can be a great way to customize your diet, but you must take care to be mindful of your body and its reactions to a carb free diet. Many ketogenic diets limit carb intake to 40-60 carbs per day. Maintaining this structure for 5-7 days will allow ketones to be released slowly into the bloodstream. While adhering to this diet structure is a safe way to burn fat and induce a ketogenic state, it is not for beginners.

So the Ketogenic diet is probably the most effective to achieve healthy weight loss, but should be reserved for those who have experience with intermittent fasting and other dieting experiences. Let's take a quick look at some ketogenic keywords for reference;

Ketosis

A natural metabolic process induced but lack of quick energy to be used, instead the body turns to stored fat energy to burn.

Ketones

Acids that are released during a ketosis state, if left unregulated the ketones can turn the blood too acidic, causing health issues.

Ketoacidosis
Life-threatening illness induced by having blood that is overly acidic due to the release of ketones during ketogenic states. Often a problem for people suffering from diabetes.

We see that ketogenic diets require strict attention to detail and preferably some fasting experience before practicing. The diet can do wonders for improving the state of your health, but be aware that people with blood pressure problems or diabetes should not practice this diet.

Overview

We find a pattern in the ideal diets for an intermittent fasting routine. Fresh, unprocessed ingredients and a colorful variety of foods are integral to all of these diets. When choosing a diet be sure to find one that is going to still be enjoyable for your to eat. Even the slightest alteration to your typical diet will yield great results. By cutting out excess sugars and processed foods you will notice more energy and overall a better physical feeling. Feeling good physically will lead to feeling good mentally. Even without an intermittent fasting practice, an overhaul of your diet can change your life. Combined with an intermittent fasting routine a balanced diet can be a transformative practice, improving all aspects of your life.
We have now connected the dot on the relationship between intermittent fasting and a balanced diet. There is no question

that intermittent fasting is a safe and effective stepping stone to our desired goals. The scientific studies cannot be ignored, fasting helps in the regulation of the organ function that affect weight loss, all the while being able to induce states that actually burn reserved fat cells. Combined with a casual exercise practice, healthier eating patterns and positive perspective, we can be on our way on our transformative path. And if this isn't enough to induce a sense of motivation, these practices typically have a positive impact on the environment and can inspire others to develop their awareness of their diets and healthy choices.

We now continue on our transformative path to our weight loss or detox goals. Picture yourself with your new knowledge on the science and practice of intermittent fasting, we've considered exercise and fasting techniques, we have seen the balanced diets. Let's now look at a comprehensive guide to fasting with the various techniques mentioned above.

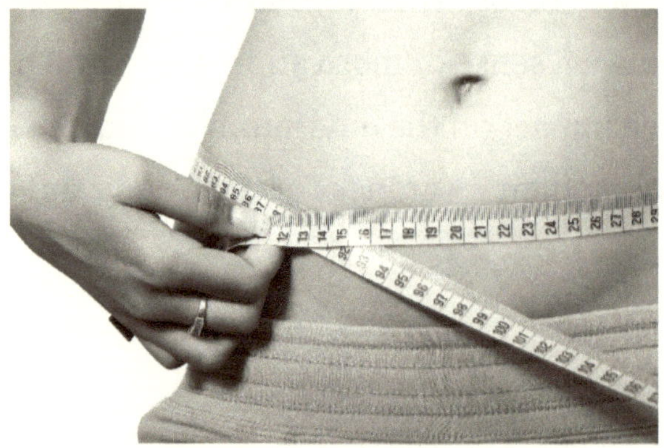

(Weight loss results on belly)

Chapter 6: Step by Step Intermittent Fasting Program

Now that we have educated ourselves in the basics of intermittent fasting and the suitable diets, we can begin developing a fasting routine to introduce into our lives. When choosing a fasting technique we must consider our goals. Are we seeking to shed some weight? Or are we trying to transform our entire life for the better? Visualize your goals and keep them in mind throughout your practice.

We now that an intermittent fasting routine can transform our lives and the world around us. With this great power we must choose wisely how we approach our new intermittent fasting routine. For the guides below we will list each intermittent fasting technique and a seven day plan for each to get you started. These guides are loose guideline to help you develop your own customized routine. Start with these guides and then customize it to your liking to get the best results. We will treat these guides as if the reader is a complete beginner.

For many people you will want to have a preparatory week before your planned fasting week. This week is designed to help your body ease into the intermittent fasting routine in the safest way. You may skip the preparatory week if you feel comfortable approaching your new practice. Let's discuss the preparatory week and how it would look to a beginner.

Preparatory Week

As you approach your first intermittent fasting week we need to prepare the body for the new routine. This preparatory week is highly recommended for those who feel that their diet is incredibly unhealthy or unbalanced. The preparatory week will help you adapt to your new diet and fasting practice. Sometimes people experience a shock to their body when they abruptly adopt an intermittent fasting routine, the preparatory week aims to avoid this shock.

Consider you last week of meals. We need to examine our diet and think about the necessary changes you need to make to improve our diet. Make a list of the foods you can keep in your diet and a list of foods that need to be eliminated. During your next grocery shopping trip you need to be strict and replace the eliminated ingredients with healthier options. If it helps, make a seven day list of the meals you will have for your preparatory week. Choose a diet from the 'diet' chapter and adhere to it. Perhaps you want to try a vegetarian diet, or maybe you are going to try the Mediterranean diet. However you choose to alter your diet, be honest with yourself and be open minded to new foods.

Our preparatory week will begin on Sunday and go to Saturday. The Sunday of your preparatory week you will go grocery shopping for your new diet plan. Make a list and stick to it. If it helps you can use meal prepping to organize your diet. This practice is done by making your meals for the week all at once and storing them to be eaten throughout the week. Let's say you choose the Mediterranean diet. A solid shopping list for Mediterranean inspired meals for our preparatory week may look like this:

- Avocados
- Olives
- Squash
- Spinach
- Onion
- Tomatoes
- Broccoli
- Cucumber
- Carrots
- Apples
- Bananas
- Berries
- Goat Cheese
- Greek Yogurt
- Local Honey
- Almonds

- Garbanzo Beans
- Black Beans
- Whole Grain Pasta
- Whole Grain Breads
- Rosemary
- Oregano
- Basil
- Extra Virgin Olive Oil
- Salmon
- Tuna
- Chicken
- Red Wine
- Chocolate

This list can of course be altered, it is just a loose guideline for healthful ingredients. For this preparatory week we should eat at the typical times that you normally eat, only with the new meal plan. Let's take a look at what a standard day may look like using the shopping list above.

Breakfast

A breakfast for a Mediterranean diet is typically light and sweet. Have plenty of water in the morning, and coffee or tea if you enjoy caffeine. Breakfast sets the tone for the day so it is best to keep it light and balanced. Plenty of carbs and sugars for quick energy, and easy on-the-go options if you have rushed mornings.

Some options for breakfast may include toast and jam, toast and avocado, yogurt with honey or fruit smoothies.

Lunch

For lunches during our prep week we will have another light meal. THe middle of the day is perfect for some quick energy to help you finish your work shift or errands. Smoothies are great for busy days and some other options include;

- Whole Grain Tuna Sandwich with potato side
- Whole Grain bread with Peanut Butter with Yogurt and Honey side
- Veggie Wrap with Whole Grain Tortilla
- Chicken Wrap With Whole Grain Tortilla
- Chicken Soup with Whole Grain Crackers

Dinner

The Mediterranean dinner is often comprised of a large meal with plenty of bread and other carbs. Breads are often baked fresh and served with salads or herbs. Dinner is a time to indulge and celebrate, perhaps red wine is in order, or a sweet dessert, among other meals:

- Salmon with Steamed Greens and Potatoes.
- Whole Grain Pasta with Vegetables and Red Sauce
- Grilled Lamb with Potatoes and Vegetables

- Homemade Pizza with Goat Cheese and Vegetables
- Grilled Chicken Salad and Vegetables

Desserts and Snacks

Snacks and desserts are great for cheat days or as a reward for a successful fasting week. Do not over indulge in these treats and quick snacks, but use them sparingly as a way to break up the monotony of fasted meals. Some healthy snacks and desserts may include;

- Granola with Yogurt and Honey
- Fruit salad
- Whole Grain baked goods, muffins and sweet breads
- Nuts and Seeds
- Peanut Butter with apples

With the simple guide above you should easily complete a week of healthy meals in preparation for your first intermittent fasting week. Take note of how your body reacts to the new foods, some people may feel that the need to have two weeks of prep time to let their body adjust. Not everyone will have the same reactions so be mindful of your body and its needs. Be thinking of your fasted week as it approaches. Are you nervous? Do you feel comfortable with the new diet and practice? Ask the difficult questions and do not be ashamed if you are nervous or need extra prep time.

First Intermittent Fasting Week

Your preparatory week is coming to an end and you're ready to start your first fasting week. As the weekend comes close we need to get groceries for the fasted week. Choose which intermittent fasting technique you wish to use from the guides below and buy your groceries accordingly. Have all the groceries you need for the first week so you will not have to worry about it when the week comes.

You may want to keep your Mediterranean diet plan, but you may also change your diet as you wish. For the guides below we will be using a variety of meal plans, but all of them are going to be healthful and balanced. Follow the weekly guides closely or use them as a loose guide. We will use Saturdays as cheat days for all the following guides, feel free to change this as well. For each fasting technique you will want to have your groceries and meals planned meticulously to avoid any temptation to grab fast foods or junk foods. Be strict in your convictions and be disciplined as we continue.

You've taken the time during your prep week to consider the intermittent fasting techniques that may suit your needs. Find the chosen technique below and follow the guide for your first week of fasting. After this initial week you can make the necessary changes to fit the diet into your life and make the customizations needed to get optimal results.

5:2

For this guide we will choose the popular 5:2 technique. This technique is great for beginners as it allows plenty of room to test the waters for your intermittent fasting practice.

You have chosen the 5:2 technique, this technique asks that we restrict caloric intake on two of the days this week. Choose two days that are fitting for your schedule. For this particular guide we will choose two days that are not together in the week. We will restrict calorie intake to less than 500 for these two days. For this guide let's choose Tuesday and Thursday.

You have chosen your fast days, your groceries are stocked and your mind is ready to start your brand new intermittent fasting practice. Let's start our 5:2 week.

Sunday
The first day of our fasted week arrives and you wake up prepared and excited. Treat this day like a typical day of meals. Breakfast may consist of a whole grain bagel with light cream cheese. Have some fruit on the side, coffee or tea and plenty of water to drink.

Lunch time comes around and we will have light lunch of chicken salad on whole grain bread, with yogurt and fruit for dessert. A smoothie can accompany this light meal and plenty of water to drink. Dinner time arrives and we've almost completed and pretty casual Sunday. For dinner we can have chicken, potatoes and a preferred vegetable on the side

Monday

Monday will set the tone for the rest of the week as we approach our first fasted day. Are you excited? How does your body feel? Be mindful and listen close to your body.

Let's have a vegetarian meal for breakfast. Two eggs and toast with a glass of orange juice is perfect to start our week. Coffee or tea if needed and plenty of water.

A special note about caffeinated beverages: Caffeine is a favorite of many people to start their day. When it comes to fasting these beverages are fine to ingest since there is no calorie content. But be warned that on an empty stomach caffeine can have more intense effects. If you are sensitive to caffeine drink coffee or tea on an empty stomach is not recommended. If you find that your stomach gets upset when drinking caffeinated beverages during fasts, then cease to ingest the drinks.

Lunch approaches and we will have a light lunch in preparation of our first fasted day. Large leafy green salad with plenty of vegetables and your favorite dressing. Fruit smoothies add a nice sweet finish with this meal, add a protein supplement that is plant based, such as pea or hemp.

Dinner for this evening will vegetarian stir fry consisting of rice, chicken and vegetables. This will be a nice filling meal before a fast day. As you prepare for bed take note of how your body feels and listen close as you prepare your mind for the fast day tomorrow. Are you feeling confident? Do you have your 500 calories planned for tomorrow? Get some rest and be excited for your first fasted day, and the first day of your new life.

Tuesday

Today is the first intermittent fasting day. Today we will keep our caloric intake to below 500 calories. You can choose to spread these calories over the course of the day or have them in one meal. For this guide we will essentially skip breakfast, drink plenty of water and have unsweetened coffee or teas. You may add lemon to your water if you wish.

Lunchtime arrives and you may be feeling the effects of the fast. Listen to your body and note any distinct feelings. Lunch may also be skipped but for this guide we will be having a 200 calorie snack. Avocado toast will be a flavorful and filling meal for our fasted day. One whole avocado on two slices of toast. Season with salt, pepper and lemon.

For dinner we will have a meal that is slightly more caloric than lunch, comprised of a 300 calorie meal. Chicken quesadillas with pico de gallo are a great meal for this evening. As you have your dinner take note of how you feel. Are you fatigued? Do you feel lighter? Is there any discomfort? Be mindful as you finish dinner.

You have completed your first fasted day. As you get ready for bed congratulate yourself and take note of how you feel. This simple fasted day will be repeated on Thursday.

Wednesday

For breakfast on this day we will have two eggs with a side of whole grain toast, not unlike Monday. We can add a smoothie as well for a filling snack. Coffee and tea if needed and drink plenty of water with lemon added if you wish.

At lunch we will have a leafy green salad, with almonds and vegetables. Have fruit on the side for sweetness and of course plenty of water to drink.

For dinner we will have a chicken sandwich with a side salad. This nice light dinner will be great to ease into our second fasted day tomorrow. We are now officially half way through our first fasted week. Are you ready for tomorrow's fast?

Thursday

This day will be identical to Tuesday. The second fasted day starts by again skipping caloric intake for breakfast, opting to have only water with lemon or a caffeinated beverage.

Another snack sized lunch of 200 calories. Have a medium sized salad with our preferred dressing and plenty of vegetables. Salads and veggies are excellent for restricted calorie days since they have a low calorie count.

Dinnertime approaches and we will have a slimming meal of a chicken breast, not breaded. Add a side salad and water to drink. This meal will be the end of our second fasted day. How are you feeling? Be proud as you get to bed as you have completed your second fasting day and essentially your first intermittent fasting week.

Friday

You awake this day with your first intermittent fasting week behind you. How are you feeling? Are you excited about the first weekend of your new life? For breakfast eat what you typically do in the mornings. A veggie omelet with hash browns and toast will be on the menu for this guide. Coffee, tea, juice and water for drinks.

Lunch can be a typical lunch that you enjoy. Try a grilled chicken sandwich with whole grain crackers and cheese for a snack. Water or a smoothie to drink. Take note of how your body is reacting to a day full of typical meals. Do you get more full quicker? Are you feeling confident that you can maintain a fasted week next week? Or will you maybe choose every other week to fast? Customize your practice as you wish. Maybe you will try a more challenging intermittent fast for next week.

For dinner this Friday we will prepare pasta and tomato sauce with bread and salad on the side. This wholesome, calorie dense meal will no doubt be very filling. Celebrate your success with a dessert or glass of red wine. Look back on your week and determine what you could change about the meals or fasting technique. Perhaps this technique is perfect for you. Whatever you choose to do next week be proud that you have successfully began your new life!

Saturday
Saturday is cheat day so eat whatever you like. Do not take advantage of cheat days, but use them to relax and prepare for your next week of intermittent fasting. Do your grocery shopping for next week today, go out to eat with friends or celebrate in other ways.

16:8

The 16:8 diet is slightly more challenging than the 5:2 technique. For the 16:8 we are asked to fast for sixteen hours each day with an eight hour window to eat as much as we like. We must make it a point not to take advantage of the eight hour window in an unbalanced way. This window needs to be used to get nutrient rich foods rather than indulging in unhealthy meals.

Since there is just an eight hour window to eat we must choose where this window is placed during the day. We must eat during the same window each day, so if the intake window is in the morning then we need to keep it in the morning each day. For this guide we will choose an eight hour window in the evening from 2 p.m. to 10 p.m. Feel free to choose an eight hour window that fits into your schedule, even if it's not in the evening.

Sunday

Assuming you have gathered your needed groceries for the week, this morning is going to be casual and relaxed as we prepare for our 16:8 intermittent fasting week. Since we are placing our intake window in the evening there will be no breakfast this morning. Drink plenty of water and have an unsweetened caffeine drink.

Depending on what time you eat lunch, this meal may be skipped as well. If your lunch time falls within the 2 p.m. to 10 p.m. timeframe then you may have a lunch meal. For this guide we will skip lunch and only have water with lemon for lunch. If you are feeling faint or uncomfortable have a granola bar handy just in case you need some quick energy. There is no shame in having a small snack, your safety comes first with the intermittent fasting practice.

As the midday comes to an end, you may be feeling quite hungry. As long as your selected timeframe has started you may want a late afternoon snack to get you through to dinner. As our intake window approaches you may want to be preparing your meal. For your first intake window let's get it light and have seared salmon with lemon, A side of potatoes and a side salad. We see that this meal it pretty light, but if you like you can double up on portions, this intake window is open to any and all foods, but be responsible.

As you get ready for bed take note of your body's reactions to the new intermittent fasting routine. Did the dinner meal fill you up? Are you prepared for the next day of fasting? Be sure to keep your intake window as the only time you ingest foods. Get some rest and be ready for tomorrow.

Monday

Take note of how your body feels this morning. Since our intake window is in the evening we will be skipping breakfast. Drink plenty of water and have an unsweetened caffeinated beverage if you wish.

Lunch will once again be skipped to be replaced with plenty of water. Pay close attention to your body and if you feel any discomfort ingest a small amount of calories, your safety comes first always.

As dinner time arises you are able to intake calories. Have a quick snack as you prepare dinner. This evening's meal can be anything you like. Try baking a lasagna filled with veggies like eggplant, zucchini and squash. A side salad and whole grain bread will round out this meal nicely.

Tuesday

Again, be aware of how your body feels this morning. Since our intake window is in the evening we will be skipping breakfast. Drink plenty of water and have an unsweetened caffeinated beverage if you wish.

Lunch will once again be skipped to be replaced with plenty of water. Pay close attention to your body and if you feel any discomfort ingest a small amount of calories, your safety comes first always.

As dinner time arises you are able to intake calories. If you wish, have a quick snack as you prepare dinner. This evening we will have chicken tacos with tortilla chips and salsa.

Wednesday

You have made it halfway through your first intermittent fasting week, take note of how your body feels this morning and be mindful of any adverse reactions. Since our intake window is in the evening we will be skipping breakfast once again. Drink plenty of water and have an unsweetened caffeinated beverage if you wish.

Lunch will once again be skipped to be replaced with plenty of water. Pay close attention to your body and if you feel any discomfort ingest a small amount of calories, your safety comes first always.

As dinner time arises you are able to intake calories. Have a quick snack as you prepare dinner. For tonight we will have a veggie stir fry with carrots, broccoli, zucchini and tofu or chicken. You have officially made it half way through your first intermittent fasting week, congratulate your self.

Thursday

Entering the second half of your first week, take note of how your body feels and take any necessary changes seriously. Since our intake window is in the evening we will be skipping breakfast. Drink plenty of water and have an unsweetened caffeinated beverage if you wish.

Lunch will once again be skipped to be replaced with plenty of water. Pay close attention to your body and if you feel any discomfort ingest a small amount of calories, your safety comes first always.

As dinner time arises you are able to intake calories. Have a quick snack as you prepare dinner. For dinner tonight we will have whole grain grilled cheese with homemade tomato soup.

Friday

You have made it to the end of the week, take note of how your body feels this morning, any discomfort should be noted. Do you feel lighter? Are you confident in your ability to maintain a consistent intermittent fasting practice? Since out intake window is in the evening we will be skipping breakfast again. Drink plenty of water and have an unsweetened caffeinated beverage if you wish.

Lunch will once again be skipped to be replaced with plenty of water. Pay close attention to your body and if you feel any discomfort ingest a small amount of calories, your safety comes first always.

As dinner time arises you are able to intake calories, this is the final meal before cheat day. Have a quick snack as you prepare dinner, we will be having a burger of your choice. Turkey or venison are some of the more healthy choices. Maybe you want to try a vegetarian patty. Add a side of homemade French fries and congratulate yourself on your successful fasting week.

Saturday

So you have made it through your first intermittent fasting week. How do you feel? Do you plan to keep up the 16:8 technique? Or do you want to change it up? Today you may eat whatever you like, have a dessert to celebrate, or even grab a slice of pizza from a local shop. Prepare for your next fasting week and make the necessary changes you wish to make to fit the practice into your schedule.

Warrior

This technique is more akin to a diet rather than a fasting plan. Nonetheless we it is a great way to rebuild our relationship with our diet and food in general. The Warrior diet plan asks that you only have one meal a day at the same time each day, you are allowed to snack throughout the day, but these snacks must be raw and unprocessed.

For our guide we will be having our full meal in the evening with snack sized portions of raw foods at breakfast and lunch. Feel free to customize this as you wish.

Sunday

You awake ready for your new intermittent fasting routine. Since the warrior diet requires only one full meal a day we are only able to snack for breakfast. Have some granola and honey or skip breakfast altogether and only have coffee or tea. Drink plenty of water this morning and continue on with your day.

Lunch will also consist of a snack sized portion of food. Choose seeds or nuts, or raw veggies and fruits. Of course, have plenty of water to stay hydrated.

As dinner time arises you are able to intake calories. Have a quick snack as you prepare dinner. This evening's meal can be anything you like.

Monday

Since the warrior diet requires only one full meal a day we are only able to snack for breakfast. Have some granola and honey or skip breakfast altogether and only have coffee or tea. Drink plenty of water this morning and continue on with your day. Take note of how your body feels today, are you confident in your abilities to finish the week? Are there any noticeable reactions?

As midday approaches you are full swing into your first intermittent fasting week. Lunch will also consist of a snack sized portion of food. Choose seeds or nuts, or raw veggies and fruits. Of course, have plenty of water to stay hydrated.

As dinner time arises you are able to intake calories. You may have a quick snack as you prepare dinner, but don't spoil your appetite. This evening's meal will consist of a huge salad of leafy greens and unbreaded chicken, fill up and then get ready for bed. Take note of your body's reactions to the new routine and be prepared to do it all over again tomorrow.

Tuesday

This day will look identical to the previous days since the warrior diet requires only one full meal a day. We will be having a snack sized portion for breakfast. Trail mix or granola will suffice, or skip breakfast altogether and only have coffee or tea. Drink plenty of water this morning and add lemon if you'd like.

Lunch will also consist of a snack sized portion of food as well. Choose nuts or a trail mix of seeds and dried berries, or raw veggies and fruits. Plenty of water to fill up on and you're on with your day.

The evening arises and I'm sure you're ready to eat. Have a quick snack while you are preparing dinner and perhaps a drink of fruit juice or red wine. This evenings meal will be baked potatoes topped how you choose with a lean meat like venison steak. Again, this evening look back at your day and analyze how your body felt and how your energy levels were. Get some rest and be ready for tomorrow.

Wednesday
Breakfast today will be like the previous days. Have some trail mix or snack sized portions of fruit or skip breakfast altogether and only have coffee or tea. Fill up on water with lemon and carry on with the morning.

More snack sized portions for lunch, the ever reliable trail mix or mixed nuts. AS you approach the middle of the week ask yourself if this fast is working for you. Do you enjoy this routine? Does your body seem to be functioning properly? Be honest and listen to your body as you continue your day.

Dinner time arrives and you're certainly ready for a meal. Have an appetizer of tortilla chips and salsa while you prepare a vegetarian burrito. Stuff full of beans, cheese, rice and your preferred veggies.

Thursday

You have successfully made it half way through your first intermittent fasting week! How are you feeling this morning? Another snack portion for breakfast, an apple and some peanut butter or skip breakfast altogether and only have coffee or tea. Fill up on water and continue you with your morning.

Lunch will be the same as previous days, have a snack sized portion of peanut butter on a slice of bread or tortilla. And as always, drink plenty of water to stay hydrated.

Now that the evening is approaching you can have your big meal. Feel free to have a snack while you b prepare a chicken breast with cheesy rice on the side. Have dinner rolls or other bread as well.

Friday

Your final day of the warrior week has arrived. How are you feeling? Is your body adjusting to the new routine of only one meal a day? Breakfast today will be no different than the rest of the week, have a snack sized portion or skip breakfast altogether and only have coffee or tea. Drink plenty of water this morning and continue on with your day.

Lunch will be similar to the rest of the week, a small, snack sized portion of raw foods. The home stretch is before you, once the evening comes around you will be finished with your first intermittent fasting week. Of, and be sure to drink plenty of water in the meantime.

The evening has come and you've officially completed your first fasting week. Give yourself a pat on the back for your success. Take note of how rewarding it feels to finish this week. How do you feel mentally and physically? Are you happy? Do you feel fulfilled? This evenings dinner can be whatever you like, but keep it on the healthy side and save indulgences for tomorrow's cheat day.

Saturday

This is cheat day so do as you wish with your meals. Feel free to have a dessert or go out to eat with friends or loved ones. Keep in mind your next fasting week, you will need to plan properly and gather your groceries on this day.

OMAD

This diet is the 'one meal a day' plan. It is similar to a warrior diet but there is no intake at all during the fasted window. OMAD means just that, only one meal a day. You are required to only ingest food for one sitting. No snacking just water or non-caloric drinks. This will be slightly more challenging than the warrior diet.

Sunday

You awake ready for your new intermittent fasting routine. The OMAD diet requires only one full meal a day we are to skip breakfast altogether and only have coffee or other non-caloric drinks. Drink plenty of water this morning and continue on with your day.

Lunch will also consist of only water with lemon. There is no calorie intake for this meal.

As dinner time arrives you are able to intake calories. Be mindful of your body and listen closely. Cook a hearty meal of a lean meat and potatoes, accompanied by a salad. Remember you can only eat at this time so be sure to fill up.

Monday

Since the OMAD diet requires only one full meal a day we must skip breakfast altogether and only have coffee or tea. Other non-caloric drinks are allowed as well. Drink plenty of water this morning and continue on with your day.

As midday approaches you are full swing into your first intermittent fasting week. Lunch will also consist of only water and lemon. Be sure to drink plenty of water and listen to your body.

As dinner time arises you are able to intake calories. This evening's meal will consist of a huge salad of leafy greens and grilled chicken, eat as much as you like and then get ready for bed. Take note of your body's reactions to the new routine and be prepared to do it all over again tomorrow.

Tuesday

This day will look identical to the previous days since the OMAD diet requires only one full meal a day. We will skip breakfast altogether and have non-caloric drinks. Drink plenty of water this morning and add lemon if you'd like.

Lunch will also be skipped today and replace with plenty of water to fill up on. Add lemon if you like and look forward to your evening meal coming soon.

As the evening arrives you are surely ready for a meal. Keep in mind that you can only eat during this one setting so be sure to get your fill. Prepare spaghetti with tomato sauce tonight. Add turkey meat balls and have salad or bread for an appetizer.

Wednesday

Breakfast today will be like the previous days. We will need to skip out o nany caloric intake and only have non-caloric drinks. Fill up on water with lemon and carry on with the morning.

You are officially half way through your first intermittent fating week. How is your body adjusting to the new practice? Do you feel like you have more or less energy? Skip lunch again today and only have water with lemon. Congratulate yourself on making it this far and move on with the day.

Dinner time arrives and you're certainly ready for a meal. We will prepare salmon with asparagus and lemon tonight. Fill up with a dessert of your choice and be sure not to overindulge.

Thursday

You are fully immersed in your fast at this point in the week, be aware of your body and take note of how you feel. We will skip breakfast altogether and only have coffee or tea for breakfast. Fill up on water and continue you with your day.

Lunch will be the same as previous days, only consisting of water with lemon or herbal teas. You may be really feeling the effects of the fasted week by this point. Stay positive and keep your mind busy. Dinnertime is coming soon.

The evening approaches and you're ready for a full meal. Since we have missed out on so many breakfasts this week we are going to treat ourselves with breakfast for dinner. Prepare an omelet with spinach and tomato. Add toast with jam for a side and maybe even hash browns. Only one more full day to go and you've completed your first fasting week.

Friday

Be very aware of how your body feels this morning. It is the final day of your OMAD fast and you need to look back at the week and recall all the experiences you have had. This morning we are once again going to skip breakfast altogether and only have coffee or tea. Drink plenty of water this morning and continue on with your day.

Lunch will be similar to the rest of the week, consisting of only water with lemon or other non-caloric drinks. Only a few hours left until you've finished the week. Be strong and look forward to the upcoming meal.

The evening has come and you've officially completed your first fasting week. Give yourself a pat on the back for your success. Take note of how challenging the week has been. Are you fatigued? Do you feel like you could complete another week of the OMAD diet? For dinner tonight have a meal of your choosing and celebrate your new path of transformation. Save room for tomorrow's cheat day and consider your next step on the intermittent fasting path.

Saturday

This is cheat day so do as you wish with your meals. Feel free to have a dessert or go out to eat with friends or loved ones. Keep in mind your next fasting week, you will need to plan properly and gather your groceries on this day.

Spontaneous

The spontaneous method of intermittent fasting is just that, spontaneous. You will fast whenever it is convenient or simply when you feel like a restricted calorie day. This method does not require a day by day guide but will need some discussion.

When spontaneously choosing fasting days you will find that the days will seem to choose themselves. You have a busy day and find that you haven't eaten and it's evening time, might as well just call it a fast and get ready for bed. Many new parents find themselves in these situations, may as well call it a fast day and get some rest. These days can come in many forms, maybe you just don't feel hungry some days, or perhaps you just feel like only eating raw foods another day. There are endless ways to approach this method.

This method does not really require structure or discipline, so it may not be as valuable to some people. But for those who are less serious about transformation and just want to dabble in the practice of intermittent fasting, this method is very useful. If you have a busy schedule or cannot commit to a week-long fast, try the spontaneous method and fast when it's perfectly convenient for you.

Alternating

This method of intermittent fasting requires you to fast every other day. This is pretty self-explanatory, but what kind of fast should you choose for the fasted days? Take some inspiration from the other fasting techniques to decide what type of fast you will do every other day. For the guide below we will choose to fast completely on the fasting days. This means that we will not consume calories on fasted days, only water or non-caloric drinks. If you wish to add some calorie content to these days try keeping it under 500 – 600 per day.

Sunday

Your first day arrives and you awake wholly prepared, this Sunday we will be having our normal eating schedule, but be prepared for tomorrow's fasted day. Contemplate your upcoming week this morning, but otherwise treat this morning like any other. Eat your typical meals or try a vegetarian day to switch it up.

Lunch time will be typical of our normal eating schedule. Have a balanced lunch that is colorful and not too heavy. Keep your fasting week ahead at the forefront of your mind.

As dinner arrives you get one last meal before our first fasted day of the week. Have a nice light meal, full of vegetables and fruits. Keep the calorie count low in anticipation of the fasted day tomorrow.

Monday

Today is our first fasted day. For all of your meals today you will only be having water. You may add lemon to your water, but other than that it is recommended that you only ingest water. Keep a granola bar or some source of quick energy handy just in case you need it. If you feel faint or lightheaded eat some of your snack. Always keep your safety the first priority when it comes to fasting.

For Tuesday through Friday you can keep this alternating method going. Tuesday will look like Sunday. Wednesday will be another fasted day like Monday. You will eat in Thursday, like Sunday, but fast in Friday. Saturday will once again be a cheat day where you can do as you like.

Notes on Cheat Days

We have mentioned cheat days throughout this entire book. Cheat days are self-explanatory; you get to eat whatever you wish and indulge in your favorite foods. This behavior may be frowned upon in many fitness circles but with our intentions with this book we accept cheat days as crucial in rebuilding a balanced and enjoyable relationship with our bodies. There is nothing bad about rewarding yourself on a cheat day. Take this day and go out to eat with friends or have a couple of alcoholic beverages, this day is yours to do as you wish.

This being said, we must respect our cheat days for what they are. Not only is this a day where you are able to cheat, but it is also a test of your self-control and dedication to your health. Can you easily spend a day indulging in your favorite snacks and jump back on the intermittent fasting path the next day? Cheat days are fun and rewarding, but is they are taken advantage of you may disrupt your entire practice. This is not ideal, and in fact defeats the purpose of all our hard work in this book. So here we accept cheat days as a welcome aspect of intermittent fasting. Trying to build a positive and enjoyable relationship with food is difficult, but shouldn't be practiced without joy. Choose designated cheat days assigned well ahead of time, like the third Saturday of each month for example. Some may want to have randomly selected cheat days. However you choose to spend cheat days, take the time to enjoy them wisely and include them in the relationship we are attempting to build with our diet and our bodies.

As we move on we need to consider what we have learned. The ancient history of fasting has validated it as an effective practice, the scientific backing helps as well, but has yet to reach a unanimous conclusion on its safety. So fasting as a health practice is performed safely throughout our society but what about combined with other healthy practices? Exercise and physically stressful activities need to be covered now.

Chapter 7: Fasting and Exercise

We have seen that there are many reasons someone may adopt an intermittent fasting routine. Weight loss, spirituality, detox and overall health are the key reasons. Another crucial aspect of health is physical activity. A lot of people feel that they are not able to develop an exercise practice. Their bad habits of using all their free time indulging in junk foods or alcohol leads to patterns that are difficult to change.

 The fast paced society and demanding work schedules that our world is based on often make it tough to start and maintain a balanced exercise routine. Most people hold the common misconception that you must have a gym membership to truly get into shape. This just isn't true. Simply taking walks, stretching and aerobic exercises go a long way to keep the body in shape, especially for beginners just starting out on an exercise practice.

Hiking through the woods, yoga and walking are great examples of low intensity exercises that make a huge difference on your path of transformation. These exercises are not just simple to perform, they are free and can be done anyplace. These low energy movements are also ideal for an intermittent fasting routine. Just fifteen to twenty minutes a day of these exercises can help keep your body in check.

Exercise has the support of science on its side as well. It has been shown to reduce stress and help fight weight gain. Most anyone who exercises regularly will know that it makes you feel great, physically and mentally. In general, getting up and getting the blood moving is key to maintaining a healthy lifestyle. Exercise and its ability to reduce the chances of weight gain cannot be ignored. The stress relief that you receive during an exercise routine is often noticeable during or soon after the practice. The most simple routines and casual exercises can change your life dramatically.

Exercise Myths

There is a lot of controversy about exercising during an intermittent fasting routine. Many are concerned that burning fast reserves and releasing ketones during exercise may be detrimental to their health. There are many opinions to find online, and it can be tough to find good information through the disorganization and unfounded claims. Let's discuss some of the main points of exercise and how it can affect intermittent fasting routines.

With all the misconceptions about intermittent fasting, there are just as many pertaining to exercise. These misunderstood opinions often become full on myths that people hold true. Some of the more common misconceptions are included below.

Exercise Only Benefits Physical Health
When we find fitness programs or gyms advertising it always focuses on the physical aspects of our life that they can help. With appearance being so important in the western world, it is not surprising that exercise gets an immediate link to physical health and good looks.

Exercise is important to improve physical health, but it also affects our internal organs and mind in a positive way. Our body works as a whole system that is reliant on various parts to operate together to function correctly. Without good mental health and our organs functioning correctly our physical appearances are not as important.

You Can Only Lose Weight with Exercise
This idea is a very common mindset in the popular culture. Weight loss is affected by not only physical activity, but perspective and internal health as well. Some more recent studies have found that gut bacteria play an integral role in weight loss. And the more variety you have in your diet, the more variety of gut bacteria you have. Here is a clear link between diet and exercise.

While exercise is important to getting rid of extra pounds, our diet, emotional state and genetic health play a key role as well.

Combining all these aspects and balancing our health and well-being is the fastest and safest way to achieve our desired weight.

It is best to exercise in the Morning

As we have mentioned throughout this book, no one way is going to work for everyone. Popular fitness circles have propagated the idea of exercise in the morning being the best way to work out, but this isn't necessarily true. There is really no evidence to support that morning workouts are more effective and expecting everybody to follow the same routine is foolish.

Everyone has different ideas of succeeding and what a successful workout looks like. For one person it may be a visit to the gym overnight, for others a casual mid afternoon walk. The results will be the same regardless of the time of day, do what works best for you. You develop your own routine and don't worry if it isn't identical to the popular fitness gurus.

Exercise While Fasting

There are misconceptions about exercising during fasting days too. It may seem like a good idea to exercise when fasting to burn fat reserves quickly. 'Fasted workouts' are growing in popularity and have a huge community of support. Let's take what we know about fasting and exercise and apply them to our routine.

We know that the body will burn stored fat reserves once it uses all of its quick energy supply from sugars and carbohydrates. If we have been fasting and exhaust our quick energy then we have been relying on fat reserves for some amount of time. Exercising during this time would seem like a great way to burn more fat, but there are precautions we need to take. With very few studies dedicated to the practice of fasted workouts it is tough to know for sure how safe it is. People have found success losing weight with a fasted workout, and they advocate for the practice. But we cannot expect it to work tis way for everybody. Studies have shown that recovering from a fasted workout is easier than a workout that relies on quick energy from recently eaten foods. We have also learned that fat reserves are a cleaner and more efficient energy as well.

One important aspect of fasted exercises is their proven effects over a long period of time. Studies show that workouts during fast days help the body adapt to being active with low glycogen levels, this is the defense mechanism kicking in. This may be helpful during emergency situations, and also helps your body to use its energy much more efficiently during day to day life. These practices may not be ideal for professional athletes or other physically demanding careers, but for the normal person fasted workouts are a safe and effective path to weight loss and rebuilding a healthier relationship with their bodies and diet.

Types of Exercise

There is a wide variety of workout fads and exercise structures. From intense weight training to a short hike in the woods, exercise comes in many different forms. But what types of exercise are best for fasted exercises? To ensure our safety during these exercises we must not just improvise. We should take a look at our personal preferences and limitations, and we do not have experience with our personal exercise boundaries, then we must discover them.

Many experts have found that exercises of moderate to low difficulty are perfect for a fated workout. With this in mind we need to always consider our persona boundaries when it comes to physical assertion. For example if you haven't ingested calories for three days a workout is probably not in your near future. For most people skipping calories for one day and having a light workout is safe. Know yourself and listen to your body.

Workouts that are low impact and well within your boundaries are the best for fasted workouts. A casual jog or long hike are great options for fasting days. For those experienced with working out an intensive yoga session or light weights may be suitable for a fasted workout. Those of us with blood pressure issues or other problematic health risks should consult their physician before beginning an exercise routine. Let's take a look at some low impact exercising options for the normal person seeking to add exercise to their intermittent fasting routine.

Cardiovascular

These exercises can be broadly defined as any exercise that increases your heart rate. Cardio exercise can be done through many different activities and at many different levels of difficulty. Hiking, jogging and cycling are great examples of lower impact versions of cardio exercises. Any light to moderate cardiovascular exercise is ideal for an intermittent fasting practice.

Yoga

Imported from India and gaining popularity in the 1960s and 1970s, yoga has been a popular means of mindfulness and wellness ever since throughout the western world. The English translation of yoga means 'union'. This practice strives to unite the body and mind through a disciplined practice comprised of stretches and breathing exercises. Many people believe yoga to be a religious practice, but this is a misconception. Yoga can be adopted into any lifestyle and its beneficial results are widespread throughout many cultures. Deep stretches and deep breathing are only going to benefit any intermittent fasting routine.

As far as rebuilding our relationship with our bodies yoga is going to be one of the most efficient and effective. The practice is free and a routine can be easily developed using free information online. Combined with an intermittent fasting practice yoga can transform the body and mind in ways no other form of exercise can. In fact, many can view any exercise as a type of 'yoga. While performing any structured physical activity the mind and body are in sync, creating a union. Many people experience this as being in the zone, or a flow like state that is attained through discipline and dedication.

Thai Chi

Often associated with yoga exercises, thai chi is actually slightly different. Thai chi emphasizes the movements of the body rather than held postures or stretches. As with yoga, thai chi utilizes breathing exercises as well. This ancient exercise aims to teach you how to manipulate the energy of our bodies, and balance our being while further building our relationship with our bodies.

Being able to control your breath and balance your body will go a long way to improve your physical health and learn to control your outlook on life. It has been shown that stress is reduced when we have a positive perspective, and stress is linked to weight gain problems, not to mention very disruptive to any routine. Thai chi is recognized as one of the best means of stress reduction. For people with limited mobility thai chi is ideal as well. It is incredibly low impact and can be performed by almost anyone for free.

There are plenty of resources online or thai chi classes and groups in most areas.

Running

For an exercise that will jump start any new workout, running is ideal. This exercise benefits our entire body and increases overall stamina in incredible ways. For a fasted workout be sure not to overexert while running, this activity burns calories faster than most any other. Jogging and slower running activities are much more fitting for a limited calorie day.

Running also requires you to be able to control your breath, this is essentially an added breathing exercise that accompanies the actual running. We are seeing a pattern in beneficial activities requiring breath work. Breath is incredibly important and being able to control it is integral to living a healthy life.

Running or jogging is free and the majority of people can do it. Have a run around your neighborhood or find a trail or paved path to run.

Walking

Walking may seem less effective compared to running, but in fact walking can be just as beneficial for the mind and body. While walking may not burn calories as fast as running, it is beneficial for winding down and balancing the mind. Especially with long walk like trails or hiking areas we find a great benefit for our heart and lungs.

Having a quick walk through the neighborhood is beneficial, but studies have shown that when exercise is performed outdoors or in a natural setting that it is even more beneficial for the body. Finding a good hiking trail is not difficult in most regions. People have been known to walk for miles and miles sometimes camping overnight for days as they conquer some of the longest trails in the world. You must be in peak physical condition to perform these feats.

Intensive trial or casual stroll, walking has amazing benefits for body and mind, and of course it's completely free.

Light Weight Lifting

Weight lifting can be an awesome exercise to focus attention on certain parts of the body that need it. While lifting weights is ideal for toning muscle and building muscle, its benefits are not just for appearances. Weight lifting is great for building your strength for all parts of the body.

While certain training routines require large equipment and expertise, for a fasted workout we should keep the exercises low intensity. Light weights and more aerobic routines are ideal for intermittent fasting. Be mindful when starting a weight training practice, it is also recommended that you hire an expert to avoid injury when weigh training.

These exercises are great examples of activities that are ideal for fasted workouts, but is in no way a comprehensive list. There are many more activities that will help get your mind and body into shape. Be sure to take caution while choosing exercise for intermittent fasting routines, and to not overexert yourself. As we have mentioned throughout the book it is important that you find a routine that works for you, something that you actually enjoy. There is a tendency to just follow others in their respected routine, but we need to personalize our practice. Personalizing your exercise routine will help avoid monotony and go a long way in rebuilding heathy relationship with your body. By developing your own exercise practice that you truly enjoy, you can better maintain a confident and balanced relationship with your body. We shouldn't have to dread our workouts, or feel ashamed if we miss a gym visit to go work out. Choose activities that are enjoyable to you, if you like sports choose an low impact sport to play. If you enjoy nature, hiking or climbing may be a fitting choice. And of course some people just belong in the gym!

Within the expansive array of exercise that can be done, intermittent fasting has its distinct role in your healthy routine, but keep in mind everything that we've learned in this book. There are many things to take into consideration before adopting a fasted workout, the most important being the idea that you must listen closely to your body. If you experience any pain or discomfort during a fasted workout, then stop immediately and make sure you are okay. Educate yourself when you are making drastic changes to your health routine, and be patient when you are beginning, it's okay to ease into a practice. There are some general rules when it comes to the fasted workout, these are universal for everyone:

- Drink plenty of water, it is important to stay hydrated all the time
- Keep the workouts low impact and know your limitations
- Stop immediately if you feel pain
- Listen to your body

Not everyone will be wanting to start a new exercise routine along with a new intermittent fasting routine. Taking on two brand new practices may be overwhelming but we cannot stress the importance of physical activity enough. For detox and weight loss fasting will give you needed abilities to transform your life, but to maintain this balance we must have some sort of physical activity. Exercise works similar to fasting to heal the body and engage its natural abilities to be resilient and strong. Between the two important practices there is a wealth of knowledge and experience that cannot be attained through any other means.

We see the importance of exercise in maintaining a healthy lifestyle. If you choose not to adopt an exercise routine immediately, consider it for the next step in improving your intermittent fasting practice. Once you are comfortable with your fasting routine and are in need of a more challenging practice, add a small exercise routine or other physical activity. Physically challenging hobbies are perfect for this concept. Take on a sport, go explore the forest or find another hobby that requires physical movement.

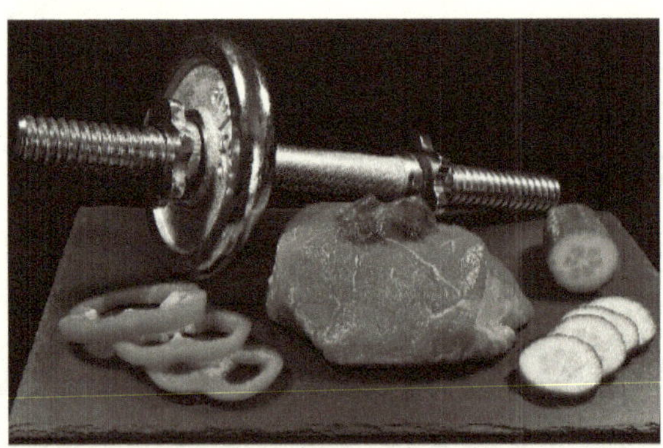

(Meat vegetables and weight)

Conclusion

Thank you for making it through to the end of *this book*, let's hope it was informative and able to provide you with all of the tools you need to achieve your goals whatever they may be. We have learned that there is no other practice that yields such great results and also has a rich history throughout many cultures and regions.

The next step is to take what you have learned in this book and further your education on intermittent fasting. Consider what your next steps will be to improve your health and balance you outlook in life. This practice is infinite in its potential to transform our lives for the better. It is safe to say that intermittent fasting can be practiced for an entire lifetime and still not be explored to the fullest extent. The mysterious nature of fasting's history along with modern science creates a balance that cannot be ignored. This practice has been an integral aspect of human living for as far back as we know

While we have learned the overall basics of intermittent fasting science, history and technique, overall health is a lifelong journey that yields many lifetime's worth of knowledge and education. We can rest assured that the science will only continue to prove the beneficial influences of intermittent fasting. There will always be sceptics and naysayers, but from experience only you as an individual actually know if the practice is right for you. Take what you've learned and continue to transform your life.

The strict and ever experimental of science aside, the intellectual and spiritual value gained from intermittent fasting is infinite. As we strive to become our desired self through these transformative practices we are essentially making a statement about our society, our culture and humanity as a whole. If we want to be the change we want to see in the world, we need to be a prime example of balance and health. The benefits fasting offers to improve the chances of longevity and positivity are invaluable.

With this very empowering notion of transformation, we must also consider the responsibility that comes along with these incredible practices. There is a responsibility to ourselves as well to others around us. This responsibility is comprised of individual aspects as well as global ones. If we are to advocate an intermittent fasting lifestyle we must be balanced examples of the practice. You may find that some people, especially online, will claim to use these practices but in fact only brag about their routine to gain popularity or get likes on their social media. While this is fine for those who simply wish to gain popularity, if we actually want to transform our relationship with our bodies and minds we need to have an honest approach to these serious practices. This honesty with yourself will go a long way to developing a positive outlook on your practice and your body.

While not all of us are aiming to ensure drastic social change, when we take on an intermittent fasting routine we are impacting our surroundings whether we know it or not. Throughout our society many people are seeking inspiration from other individuals, rather than popular companies or groups. This internet has forever changed the way we interact with each other and health is not immune to this new technology. Casual discussions with loved ones about intermittent fasting can change their whole perception on diet and health. We may not all be social justice warriors at heart, but we can make it a point to be aware and thoughtful of our peers and what they are going through on their health journeys. Be open minded toward sceptics and ridicule, and always be humble and transparent when expressing your love of intermittent fasting.

As we conclude this book we are left with a sense of an important choice to be made. How can we improve our newfound intermittent fasting practice? What does the future hold for our new routine? How will these transformations change the course of our personal lives? There are many ideas and insights offered by a mindful approach to health. As we build a new relationship with our bodies and food we must consider what else lies ahead, how in depth can this relationship go? There is only one way to find out; continue your safe intermittent fasting practice and as always listen to your body!